Master the Veterinary Technician National Examination (VTNE)

1st Edition

T0151106

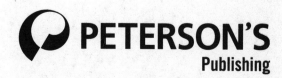

PETERSON'S

Publishing

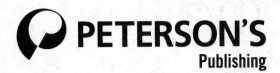

About Peterson's Publishing

To succeed on your lifelong educational journey, you will need accurate, dependable, and practical tools and resources. That is why Peterson's is everywhere education happens. Because whenever and however you need education content delivered, you can rely on Peterson's to provide the information, know-how, and guidance to help you reach your goals. Tools to match the right students with the right school. It's here. Personalized resources and expert guidance. It's here. Comprehensive and dependable education content—delivered whenever and however you need it. It's all here.

For more information, contact Peterson's Publishing, 2000 Lenox Drive, Lawrenceville, NJ 08648; 800-338-3282 Ext. 54229; or find us online at www.petersonspublishing.com.

Bernadette Webster, Director of Publishing; Jill C. Schwartz, Editor; Ray Golaszewski, Publishing Operations Manager; Linda M. Williams, Composition Manager

ISBN-13: 978-0-7689-3372-7
ISBN-10: 0-7689-3372-2

Printed in the United States of America

10 9   24 23

First Edition

Contents

PART I: A Career as a Veterinary Technician

PART II: Diagnosing Strengths and Weaknesses

Contents

PART III: Types of Questions on the Veterinary Technician National Exam (VTNE)

PART IV: Two Written Exam Practice Tests

Appendixes

Special Advertising Section

University of Medicine & Dentistry of New Jersey

Jefferson School of Population Health (Thomas Jefferson University)

Saint Louis University

St. Mary's University

The Winston Preparatory Schools

Before You Begin

OVERVIEW

- How this book is organized
- Special study features
- You're well on your way to success
- Give us your feedback
- Today's opportunities for veterinary technicians

HOW THIS BOOK IS ORGANIZED

Veterinary technician is a good career choice for individuals who love animals and want to spend their days caring for them. Veterinary technicians also often enjoy job security, good pay, and great benefits. The U.S. Bureau of Statistics reports that over the next decade, employment for veterinary technicians is expected to grow much faster than average and overall job opportunities should be excellent.

Those interested in becoming a veterinary technician must complete a two-year associate degree program accredited by the American Veterinary Medical Association (AVMA) and then take and pass a national examination, the Veterinary Technician National Examination (VTNE), which is offered in most states.

The veterinary technician career has changed significantly in recent years—from the job title itself to employment prospects. For more on this, take a look at "Today's Opportunities for Veterinary Technicians," by Kimberly Myers, Associate Professor of Veterinary Technology at the University of Cincinnati, which appears at the end of this section.

This book was carefully researched and written to help you prepare for the VTNE. The chapters in this book explain what it is like to work as a veterinary technician and review important material that is likely to appear on the VTNE. Completing the many practice exercises and practice tests in this book will help you pass this exam.

To get the most out of this book, take the time to read each section carefully and thoroughly.

- **Part I** provides an overview of a veterinary technician's job responsibilities and the places where veterinary technicians work. It offers information about the education you need to become a veterinary technician and the subjects assessed on the Veterinary Technician National Examination (VTNE), the national exam given in most states. Part I also outlines the steps you need to take to become a veterinary technician, including preparing and applying for the VTNE and becoming registered, licensed, and/or certified.

- **Part II** is a preview of the written examination. This section introduces you to the kinds of questions you will see on the VTNE, including questions about pharmacy, pharmacology, surgical preparation and assisting, laboratory procedures, animal care and nursing, anesthesia and analgesia, and dentistry and diagnostic imaging.

- **Part III** is a comprehensive overview of the types of questions you will see on the VTNE. A chapter is devoted to each subject area, or domain, on the test. Each chapter begins with a review of the subject matter to refresh your memory as to what you learned in school. At the end of each chapter are practice exercises. The multiple-choice questions in the practice exercises are just like those on the actual test. Complete the questions and study the answer explanations. You can learn a great deal from these explanations. Even if you answered the questions correctly, you may discover a new tip in the explanation that will help you answer other questions.

- When you feel that you are well prepared, move on to **Part IV**—the Practice Tests. These practice examinations contain new questions modeled after the samples provided in *Information for Candidates on the Veterinary Technician National Examination*, published by Professional Examination Services (PES), the company that administers the test, which is sponsored by the American Association of Veterinary State Boards (AAVSB). The questions on the Practice Tests in this book are not the actual questions that you will see on the exam. If possible, try to work through an entire exam in one sitting. On the actual test, you will have 4 hours to complete the exam, so allow yourself this amount of time. If you must divide your time, divide it into no more than two sessions per exam. Do not look at the correct answers until you have completed the exam. Remember, these tests are for practice, and they will not be scored. Take the time to learn from any mistakes you may make.

- The **Appendixes** offer a list of medical terms and abbreviations used on the VTNE and a list of references recommended by the American Veterinary Medical Association (AVMA). Study the abbreviations until you are sure that you know them. Consult the references if you need additional veterinary information or if you have a professional question or concern.

SPECIAL STUDY FEATURES

Master the Veterinary Technician National Examination (VTNE) is designed to be as user friendly as it is complete. To this end, it includes several features to make your preparation more efficient.

Overview

Each chapter begins with a bulleted overview listing the topics covered in the chapter. This allows you to target the areas in which you are most interested.

Summing It Up

Each chapter ends with a point-by-point summary that reviews the most important items in the chapter. The summaries offer a convenient way to review key points.

Notes

Notes highlight need-to-know information about the Veterinary Technician National Exam (VTNE), whether it is details about scoring or the structure of the question type.

Tips

Tips provide valuable strategies and insider information to help you score your best on the Veterinary Technician National Exam (VTNE).

SPECIAL ADVERTISING SECTION

At end of the book, don't miss the special section of ads placed by Peterson's preferred clients. Their financial support helps make it possible for Peterson's Publishing to continue to provide you with the highest-quality test-prep, educational exploration, and career-preparation resources you need to succeed on your educational journey.

YOU'RE WELL ON YOUR WAY TO SUCCESS

You have made the decision to become a veterinary technician and have taken a very important step in that process. *Peterson's Master the Veterinary Technician National Examination (VTNE)* will help you score high on the exam and prepare you for everything you need to know on the day of the exam and beyond it. Good luck!

GIVE US YOUR FEEDBACK

Peterson's publishes a full line of books—education exploration, career preparation, test prep, and financial aid. Peterson's publications can be found at your local bookstore and library high school guidance offices, and college libraries and career centers. Peterson's books are also available as eBooks. For more information, access us online at www.petersonspublishing.com.

We welcome any comments or suggestions you may have about this publication. Your feedback will help us make educational dreams possible for you—and others like you.

Today's Opportunities for Veterinary Technicians

by Kimberly Myers, Associate Professor of Veterinary Technology

Raymond Walters College, University of Cincinnati

When I graduated as a technician in 1977, we weren't allowed to be called veterinary technicians (we were animal technicians); there were only twenty-five accredited technician programs in the country; and there was no standard testing for technicians. Much has changed since then. In 1989, we became veterinary technicians; there are now over 160 American Veterinary Medical Association (AVMA)–accredited programs; and the Veterinary Technician National Exam (VTNE) has become a reality for most technician students.

Every state has its own Veterinary Practice Act, which defines what a veterinary technician is, regulates what he or she can do, and sets standards for its veterinary technicians, although there is very little standardization among states. One thing, however, that the majority of states do require now is passing the Veterinary Technician National Exam (VTNE). This National Board Exam consists of 200 graded questions that test your knowledge on all the veterinary information you have learned over the last two years. You are never more prepared to take the exam than right after you graduate when all of the topics you will be tested on are fresh in your mind. Do your best in your college classes, and odds are you will do well on the National Boards. That doesn't mean that there aren't things you can do to improve your chances of being successful on the VTNE. Here are a few suggestions:

- See if your school has a study skills department that assists with strategies for taking multiple-choice exams. If your school doesn't have this type of help, go online and search for "multiple-choice test strategies." There is a mountain of information that can help you reason your way to the correct answer.

- Take out your notes from your classes and review the material. Review in small sections—don't try to cram the material into a few days of studying. Even if that worked for you in college, it is unlikely to be helpful when you are reviewing two years' worth of material.

- Use study guides like the one you are reading now. These guides can be a great adjunct to your VTNE preparation. They not only test (and refresh) your knowledge base and describe the correct answers, they also explain why the incorrect answers are wrong. When using a review book, find the sections that you are having the most trouble with, and spend the most time with that material.

Today's graduates have an amazing choice of career options. Small animal clinics will remain the career path for most vet techs (at least initially), yet technicians have more opportunities than ever before to keep their jobs interesting and challenging. Every year, new veterinary technician specialties gain accreditation by the *National Association of Veterinary Technicians in America* (NAVTA). Becoming a credentialed specialist involves a lot of work, but it can keep you from burnout and make you an even greater asset to your employer. Get involved with your local, state, and national professional organizations. These associations give you a chance to network with other technicians, obtain continuing education credits, and find out what job openings are available.

One thing I want to stress is that veterinary technology is a wide-open field with no shortage of career opportunities. If you are not happy where you work, don't be afraid to change. I worked in private practice and research before I found my niche in teaching. I wasn't afraid to change, and I have never regretted any of my decisions. I hope that in thirty-five years, you will feel the same way.

Kimberly Myers is an Associate Professor in the Veterinary Technology Department at University of Cincinnati's Raymond Walters College. A teacher in the Veterinary Technology Program since 1983, Kim instructs a variety of courses including Anatomy and Physiology, Radiology, and Medical Records as well as the Preceptorship portion of the program. Kim is very involved with the Cincinnati Veterinary Technicians Association and the Ohio Association of Veterinary Technicians organizations, having held a variety of offices in each. Kim is also the faculty advisor for the student chapter of the National Association of Veterinary Technicians in America. Kim received an A.A.S. in animal health technology and a B.S. in biology from the University of Cincinnati.

A Career as a Veterinary Technician

CHAPTER 1

What Is a Veterinary Technician?

OVERVIEW

- **Where veterinary technicians work**
- **Educational requirements**
- **Veterinary Technician National Examination (VTNE)**
- **Salary and benefits**
- **Employment outlook**
- **Credentials**
- **Veterinary technician specialist (VTS)**
- **Veterinary technician societies**
- **Advancement opportunities**
- **Summing it up**

Today's pet owners want their pets to receive the best possible care. They prefer to take their pets to state-of-the-art veterinary facilities offering advanced procedures such as preventative dental care, sonograms, and EKGs. Veterinarians rely on the skills of veterinary technicians to offer pets the superior care that their owners desire.

Veterinary technicians are sometimes called *veterinary nurses* because they assist a veterinarian the way a nurse assists a physician. Veterinary technicians' duties vary depending on the type and size of the practice in which they work, but they all provide direct animal care under the supervision of a veterinarian. A veterinary technician may examine pets, take their vital statistics, administer medications and vaccinations, draw blood, prepare tissue samples, update patients' charts, and communicate with pet owners.

Veterinary technicians are part of the veterinary health-care team. They work with veterinarians, who diagnose and treat animals' diseases and injuries, prescribe medications, and perform surgeries. Veterinary technicians might also work with veterinary technologists, who perform many of the same duties but have a higher level of education. In most veterinary practices, veterinary technicians work with veterinary assistants, who perform nonmedical duties such as comforting animals, cleaning cages, and grooming dogs and cats.

To become a veterinary technician, you must complete a program accredited by the American Veterinary Medical Association (AVMA) that leads to an associate degree after two years. Before being granted a license, most states require veterinary technicians to take and pass the Veterinary Technician National Examination (VTNE). This book prepares you to take that examination.

WHERE VETERINARY TECHNICIANS WORK

The vast majority of veterinary technicians work in private veterinary practices where the veterinarian specializes in treating small animals, such as cats, dogs, and birds. Veterinary technicians also work in veterinary practices that treat large animals, emergency animal hospitals, research facilities, and zoos.

Small-Animal Practices

Small-animal veterinary practices are busy places. Veterinary technicians working in such practices have many duties. They often see a pet and its owner before the veterinarian. They might sit beside an owner to obtain and document a pet's medical history. Some veterinarians rely on veterinary technicians to initially examine the pet and check for parasites and abnormalities. Veterinary technicians might also obtain the pet's vital statistics by taking its temperature, blood pressure, and pulse rate and monitoring its breathing. A veterinary technician might also assist in restraining the pet so the veterinarian may administer medical care.

In small-animal practices, veterinary technicians perform diagnostic tests on animals and prepare animals for surgery. Diagnostic tests include drawing blood, performing urinalyses, taking and developing X-rays, and preparing tissue samples. Veterinary technicians might administer sonograms, EKGs, and dental care. They play an important role in surgery by prepping the animal and preparing and sterilizing the appropriate instruments. They may administer or assist in the administration of anesthesia. Some veterinary technicians also assist in surgery by holding an animal in a certain position or assisting the veterinarian as a surgical nurse would. After surgery, a veterinary technician monitors the animal as the anesthesia wears off. Veterinary technicians also provide nursing care to pets in intensive care. They might also assist in euthanasia.

Experienced veterinary technicians may have additional responsibilities such as training new employees and explaining a pet's condition to its owner. Such veterinarian technicians might also advise pet owners on training and housebreaking.

Large-Animal Practices

Large-animal practices treat animals such as horses and livestock. Veterinary technicians working in this type of practice have many of the same responsibilities as those working in a small-animal practice. Veterinary technicians working with large animals take their history, assess their vital signs, draw blood, and provide general nursing care. However, veterinary technicians working in this environment have additional responsibilities specifically related to large animals. They might clean hooves and perform tail and leg wraps. They may collect sterile milk samples and administer oral medication using a balling gun and a stomach tube. Veterinary technicians working with horses and livestock must be accustomed to the large-animal operating room, where they may use pulleys and restraints to position animals. In a large-animal practice, a veterinary technician may accompany a veterinarian to a farm or ranch to care for animals.

Animal Emergency Hospitals

Veterinary technicians employed at animal emergency hospitals frequently administer first aid to pets in need of immediate care. They frequently bandage wounds and assist in setting broken bones and emergency surgeries. They spend most of their time administering care to animals that are critically injured or ill. Because animal emergency hospitals are open 24 hours a day, 7 days a week, veterinary technicians work nontraditional hours.

Zoos

Veterinary technicians employed at zoos assist veterinarians in providing medical care to zoo animals. Veterinary technicians working in this environment perform many of the same duties as other techs—but they might perform them on an orangutan or alligator instead of on a dog or cat. Veterinary technicians working in large zoos may choose to specialize in either clinical care or research. Those focusing on clinical care work directly with zoo animals. Those focusing on research assist with experiments and collect data in the zoo's laboratory. Veterinary technicians at zoos usually have several years' experience and specialize in caring for exotic animals.

Biomedical Research Labs

Some veterinary technicians work in biomedical research labs at universities or pharmaceutical companies, where they assist in the care of research animals. They might also assist in the implementation of research projects.

EDUCATIONAL REQUIREMENTS

To become a veterinary technician, you need at least a two-year associate degree from a community college offering a veterinary technician program accredited by the American Veterinary Medical Association (AVMA). To date, about 160 colleges in forty-five states offer accredited veterinary technician programs. You can search for accredited colleges in your state on the AVMA's Web site, http://www.avma.org. These colleges offer veterinary technician courses in clinical and laboratory settings with live animals. The AVMA recommends that high school students interested in pursuing a career as a veterinary technician take as many science—especially biology—and math courses as possible.

> **NOTE**
> According to the U.S. Bureau of Labor Statistics, the future job outlook for veterinary technicians is better than most jobs, but veterinary technicians hoping to land a job in a zoo or an aquarium should expect stiff competition. These working environments attract many job candidates and have a very low job turnover.

The course sequence for a Veterinary Technician program at an accredited community college might look like this:

First Semester
Introduction to Veterinary Technology
Anatomy & Physiology of Domestic Animals I
Veterinary Clinical Chemistry I
Pre-Calculus
English Composition I

Second Semester
Anatomy & Physiology of Domestic Animals II
Laboratory Animal Science
Veterinary Clinical Pathology I
Basic Computer Skills
English Composition II

Third Semester

Pharmacology/Anesthesia

Principles of Medicine

Radiation Surgery/Radiology

Veterinary Clinical Chemistry II

Social Science Elective

Fourth Semester

Advanced Nursing Skills

Veterinary Clinical Pathology II

Exotic Animal Management & Nutrition

Social Science Elective

Humanities Elective

Fifth Semester

Small Animal Internship or Practicum

Sixth Semester

Large or Small Animal Internship or Practicum

DISTANCE EDUCATION PROGRAMS FOR VETERINARY TECHNICIANS

Some colleges offer distance learning veterinary technician programs to accommodate students with full-time jobs and family responsibilities. Most students enrolled in these programs are already employed by a veterinarian as a veterinary assistant and plan to eventually work for the same veterinarian as a veterinary technician.

Students in these programs do not attend formal college classes during the day. Instead, they complete multimedia courses that combine textbooks, Internet assignments, and videos. They also complete clinical exercises at their place of employment. Students typically communicate with professors via e-mail or phone, and their veterinarian serves as their proctor during examinations. They spend about 5 hours each week studying, and it may take four to five years to complete an associate degree.

If you are considering this option, be sure to choose a program that is fully accredited by the American Veterinary Medical Association (AVMA). For a list of colleges offering distance education programs for veterinary technicians, consult the AVAM's Web site, www.avma.org.

www.facebook.com/careerresource

VETERINARY TECHNICIAN NATIONAL EXAMINATION (VTNE)

After graduating with an associate degree from an accredited college, you must register to take the Veterinary Technician National Examination (VTNE), which is sponsored and updated by the American Association of Veterinary State Boards (AAVSB). You register for the test by accessing the AAVSB Web site (www.aavsb.org) and clicking the link to apply/register for the VTNE. While some states give different tests, most give the VTNE. To register, you complete an application and pay a fee. Once you have completed the VTNE registration and the AAVSB has verified that you have graduated from a veterinary technician program accredited by the American Veterinary Medical Association (AVMA), you will receive an Authorization-to-Test (ATT) letter by e-mail from Professional Education Services (PES), the company that administers the test.

Scheduling a Test Date

After you receive an ATT letter, you have to schedule a test date. The VTNE is administered at Prometric Testing Centers located around the United States and Canada. To schedule yourself for a specific test date and testing center, visit www.prometric.com/aavsb. If you have a disability and need to make other arrangements for your exam, visit the AAVSB Web site to learn about what documents you should complete and submit. As of 2010, the VTNE is administered throughout the United States and Canada three times a year. Since you have only three chances per year to take the exam, it's important that you meet the application deadlines.

Rescheduling and Withdrawing from Tests

If you have to reschedule your test date, you should contact Prometric through its Web site (www.prometric.com/aavsb) or by phone. You must reschedule no later than 12:00 p.m. two days (48 hours) before the test. If you need to withdraw from the test, visit the AAVSB site for information about withdrawing. You must withdraw from the exam no later than 12:00 p.m. two days (48 hours) before the test. You will be refunded your entire original fee except for a $50 processing fee.

If you fail to attend the exam without a valid excuse, you will lose your entire original fee, and you must reapply and pay the fee again to take the test. If you do not take the exam, but have a valid excuse, you will be refunded your entire original fee except for a $50 processing fee. For more information about which excuses are valid, visit the Prometric Web site. In addition, if your name or address changes after you have applied for or scheduled the exam, you should contact the AAVSB as soon as possible. You will be required to show identification at the testing site, and the name and address on your ID must match the name and address you registered with.

At the Testing Center

On the day of your scheduled exam, you should arrive at the Prometric Testing Center at least 30 minutes before your exam. Bring with you your ATT letter and a valid form of identification. Prometric Testing Centers accept government-issued passports, driver's licenses, and military IDs as forms of identification. At the testing site, you will be given further instructions about where in the building to go to take your exam. Because they are testing facilities where people need to concentrate, Prometric Testing Centers have specific rules you will be expected to follow while you take the exam. You can find more information about these rules on the Prometric Testing Centers Web site at www.prometric.com/aavsb.

Once you find the room where your test will be administered, take a seat in front of a computer. Before you begin your test, you will review tutorials to help you navigate the test and the other features on the screen. In addition to the test, candidates can access an online calculator, a clock that counts down the time you have remaining to complete the test, and a comment section for each test question.

> **NOTE**
>
> The Veterinary Technician National Examination (VTNE) is designed to evaluate a veterinary technician's competency to practice animal care. It is continuously updated so that the questions reflect the most recent knowledge of and practice in veterinary care.

You will have 4 hours to complete the test. The clock on your computer will help you track your time. During the test, you may take breaks, but the clock keeps running during your breaks so make sure you allow yourself enough time to complete the exam. Guessing on questions is not counted against you, so answer as many questions as you can on the VTNE. You might also consider first answering the questions you know and then going back to answer the questions you are unsure about. You may also comment on any of the questions on the VTNE using the spaces provided. Remember, however, that the test is timed, and commenting on questions will use up some of your testing time.

The Makeup of the VTNE

This examination has 225 multiple-choice questions that assess your knowledge of animal care in the following subjects, or domains:

- Pharmacy and pharmacology (14%)
- Surgical preparation and assisting (16%)
- Dentistry (8%)
- Laboratory procedures (15%)
- Animal care and nursing (24%)
- Diagnostic imaging (8%)
- Anesthesia and analgesia (15%)

Of the 225 questions, only 200 are scored; the other twenty-five are pilot questions and do not count toward your score. This book will help you review the major areas to be tested and practice answering multiple-choice questions about these subjects. Note that a chapter of this book is devoted to each domain.

Pharmacy and Pharmacology

Twenty-eight questions (14 percent) on the VTNE are about pharmacy and pharmacology. Questions in this domain assess your knowledge of these tasks:

- Preparing, administering, and/or dispensing pharmacological and biological agents (excluding anesthetics and analgesics) to comply with veterinary prescriptions
- Educating the client regarding pharmacological and biological agents (excluding anesthetics and analgesics) administered or dispensed to ensure the safety of the patient's positioning

Surgical Preparation and Assisting

Thirty-two, or 16 percent, of the questions on the VTNE are about surgical preparation and assisting. Expect to answer questions about these tasks:

- Preparing and maintaining the surgical environment, equipment, instruments, and supplies to meet the needs of the surgical team and patient

- Preparing the patient for a procedure, including surgical site scrub and patient positioning

- Functioning as a sterile surgical technician (including but not limited to tissue handling, suturing, instrument handling) to ensure patient safety and procedural efficiency

- Functioning as a circulating (nonsterile) surgical technician to ensure patient safety and procedural efficiency

Dentistry

Sixteen test questions (8 percent) are about animal dentistry. These questions are about the following tasks:

- Preparing and maintaining the environment, equipment, instruments, and supplies for dental procedures to meet the needs of the dental team and patient

- Performing or assisting with dental procedures (including but not limited to prophylactic, radiographic, therapeutic, charting) to maintain the dental health of the patient and aid in the treatment of dental disease

- Educating the client regarding dental health, including prophylactic and post-treatment care

ASSISTANT VETERINARY TECHNICIANS

The National Association of Veterinarian Assistants in America (NAVTA) recently created a certification process for schools wishing to offer a veterinary technician assistant (VTA) program. Individuals who want to become assistant veterinary technicians may be able to complete the necessary course work in high school, or they may enroll in a certificate program at a community college or via a distance-learning program. Assistant veterinary technicians perform duties such as scheduling appointments, greeting customers, and answering phones. They might also file medications and maintain inventory. They restrain animals and assist veterinary technicians in administering medical care.

Laboratory Procedures

Thirty, or 15 percent, of the questions on the VTNE are about performing laboratory tests and procedures and maintaining laboratory equipment. These questions assess your knowledge of the following tasks:

- Collecting, preparing, and maintaining specimens for in-house or outside laboratory evaluation

- Performing laboratory tests and procedures (including but not limited to serology, cytology, hematology, urinalysis, and parasitology)

- Maintaining laboratory equipment and related supplies to ensure the safety of operation and quality of results

Animal Care and Nursing

About forty-eight, or 24 percent, of the exam questions are about animal care and nursing. These questions test your knowledge of the following tasks:

- Performing and documenting initial and ongoing evaluations or physical, behavioral, nutritional, and environmental status of animals to provide for optimal animal/client safety and health

- Performing animal nursing and clinical diagnostic procedures (including but not limited to postoperative care, catheterization, wound management, blood pressure measurement, and electrocardiography) to aid in diagnosis, prognosis, and implementation of prescribed treatments

- Educating clients and the public about animal care (including but not limited to postoperative care, preventative care, zoonosis) to promote and maintain the health of animals and the safety of clients and the public

- Providing a safe, sanitary, and comfortable environment for animals to ensure optimal health care and client/personnel safety

Diagnostic Imaging

Diagnostic imaging involves taking and developing radiographs, such as X-rays and sonograms. Sixteen questions (8 percent) assess your knowledge of these tasks:

- Producing diagnostic images (excluding dental) following safety protocols for operator and patient

- Maintaining imagining equipment and related materials to ensure safety of operation and quality of results

Anesthesia and Analgesia

Approximately thirty questions, 15 percent, are about anesthesia and analgesia. These questions test your knowledge of the following tasks:

- Assisting in development of the anesthetic plan to ensure patient safety and procedural efficacy

- Implementing the anesthetic plan (including but not limited to administration, monitoring, and maintenance) to facilitate diagnostic, therapeutic, or surgical procedures

- Preparing and maintaining anesthetic equipment and related materials to ensure safety and reliability of operation

- Assessing need for analgesia and assisting in the development and implementation of the analgesic plan to optimize patient comfort and healing

- Educating the client with regard to analgesic administration and the side effects of anesthetics and analgesics to ensure the safety of the patient and efficacy of the product(s) or procedure(s)

Scoring the VTNE

After you have completed the test, you will see a pass or fail score on the computer screen. This pass or fail score is preliminary, and you will receive an official score through e-mail about three or four weeks after the exam. The VTNE is scored on a scale, which means your score will not directly tell you how many questions you answered correctly. Your raw score (the number of questions you answered correctly) is converted into a scale of 200 to 800 or a scale of 0 to 100. The type of scale your test is scored on depends on the requirements of the state or province board where your results will be sent. On the 200 to 800 scale, a score of 425 and higher is passing. On the 0 to 100 scale, a score of 70 or 75 and higher (depending on your state or province's standards) is passing.

AAVSB will send your final score to the state or province board that you indicated on your application. If you want your score transferred to a different board, you can visit the AAVSB Web site to fill out an application and pay a fee.

The VTNE is created and scored by the Professional Examination Service (PES) in conjunction with the AAVSB. The PES goes through many quality assurances to ensure your exam is scored correctly. If you want your test to be scored manually, you should contact the PES within six months of taking the exam.

SALARY AND BENEFITS

Veterinary technicians earn a salary that compares favorably to other health-care occupations requiring an associate degree. A veterinary technician's salary varies depending on the location, size of the practice, and years of experience. A veterinary technician working in a city typically earns more than one working in the country.

According to the U.S. Bureau of Labor Statistics, in 2008, most veterinary technicians earned between $23,580 and $34,960. The bottom 10 percent earned less than $19,770, and the upper 10 percent earned more than $41,490.

> **NOTE**
>
> A veterinary technician's work is rewarding, but it is also dangerous. According to the U.S. Bureau of Labor Statistics, veterinary technicians and veterinary technologists report more injuries than most other occupations. Animal bites and scratches are one reason. Lifting and carrying animals, restraining animals, and cleaning cages cause many veterinary technicians to suffer injuries.

Most veterinary practices offer veterinary technicians these benefits:

- Sick leave
- Vacation pay
- Holiday pay
- Health benefits
- 401(k) plan

Some veterinary practices also offer uniform allowances, funding for continuing education, and discounts on pet care.

EMPLOYMENT OUTLOOK

The employment outlook for veterinary technicians is extremely favorable. The U.S. Bureau of Labor Statistics expects the number of veterinary technician jobs to increase 36 percent by 2018. This is significantly higher than the national average. The number of pet owners is predicted to grow, as is the number of pet owners desiring state-of-the-art procedures such as preventative dental care. Veterinarians are expected to replace many veterinary assistants with veterinary technicians, who are better qualified to assist with or provide advanced procedures.

> **NOTE**
>
> Even during a recession, pet owners continue to provide their animals with high-quality health care. Because of this, layoffs for veterinarian technicians are extremely rare.

Furthermore, fewer than 3,800 veterinary technicians are expected to graduate from accredited programs each year, a number not high enough to meet the demand. This is very good news for those pursuing a career as a veterinary technician!

CREDENTIALS

Whether you become licensed, certified, or registered depends on the state in which you live. These terms really mean the same thing—that you have the credentials to begin working as a veterinary technician. The process of becoming credentialed is similar in all states: you must graduate from a program accredited by the American Veterinary Medical Society (AVMA) and take a test assessing your competency. This test is usually the Veterinary Technician National Exam (VTNE). Then, veterinary technicians need to apply for a license, certification, or registration with a state agency such as the State Board of Veterinary Examiners. The National Association of Veterinary Technicians in America (NAVTA; www.navta.org) refers to this process as "credentialing" because states have different names for it.

Veterinary Technician's Oath

Have you ever heard of the Physician's Oath? When physicians take this oath, they promise to make the health of their patients their first priority, honor the traditions of their profession, and respect their teachers. Veterinary technicians also have an oath of their own, in which they promise to do the following:

I solemnly dedicate myself to aiding animals and society by providing excellent care and services for animals, by alleviating animal suffering, and by promoting public health.

I accept my obligations to practice my profession conscientiously and with sensitivity, adhering to the profession's Code of Ethics, and furthering my knowledge and competency through a commitment to lifelong learning.

You can read the Veterinary Technician Code of Ethics on the Web site of the National Association of Veterinary Technicians in America (NAVTA) at www.navta.org.

VETERINARY TECHNICIAN SPECIALTIES (VTS)

Some veterinary technicians choose to specialize in an area, such as internal medicine or in the treatment of a type of animal, such as exotic, or zoo, animals. To become a veterinary technician specialist, or VTS, a veterinary technician must apply for certification with an academy. The National Association of Veterinary Technicians in America (NAVTA) recognizes these academies:

- Academy of Veterinary Dental Technicians
- Academy of Veterinary Technician Anesthetists
- Academy of Internal Medicine for Veterinary Technicians
- Academy of Veterinary Emergency and Critical Care Technicians
- Academy of Veterinary Behavior Technicians

- Academy of Veterinary Zoological Medicine Technicians
- Academy of Equine Veterinary Nursing Technicians
- Academy of Surgical Technicians
- Academy of Veterinary Technicians in Clinical Practice

Most academies require veterinary technicians to have worked in the profession for several years before applying for specialization. Veterinary technicians who want to specialize usually also have to meet continuing education requirements; for example, they may have to complete 40 hours of course work in their specialty before applying for certification in this specialty. They might also have to demonstrate a competence of advanced skills and knowledge in their specialty. Some academies require applicants to submit case logs in this specialty, which are documentations of cases they have worked. Lastly, veterinary technicians wishing to specialize may have to take and pass an examination about their specialty and submit letters of recommendation.

The American Association for Laboratory Animal Science (AALAS) offers certification to veterinary technicians working in research labs. A veterinary technician with this certification is then known as a registered laboratory technician, or RLAT. To become an RLAT, an applicant must have either an associate or a bachelor's degree along with at least two years' experience in laboratory animal science. Applicants must pass an examination testing their knowledge of animal husbandry, facility management, and animal health and welfare. To learn more about this certification, consult the AALAS *Technician Certification Handbook* (http://www.aalas.org/pdf/Tech_Cert_handbook.pdf).

VETERINARY TECHNICIAN SOCIETIES

Most veterinary technicians belong to one or more societies, which are also called associations. These societies differ from academies in that they do not offer certification. A society is a group of individuals working in a certain discipline. These individuals join the society to keep abreast of the latest industry trends, share information about their occupation, and take advantage of member discounts. Veterinary technician societies exist on the national, state, and local levels.

The National Association of Veterinary Technicians in American (NAVTA) is a national, or nationwide, society. Veterinary technicians belonging to this society take advantage of such benefits as a subscription to *The NAVTA Journal* and the *NAVTA* e-newsletter, a discount to state associations, and discounts to certain retail stores. Many states and some cities also have associations for veterinary technicians.

ADVANCEMENT OPPORTUNITIES

Veterinary technicians wishing to advance and earn a higher salary may complete a four-year program and obtain a bachelor's degree. This additional education allows them to work as veterinary technologists. Experienced veterinary technicians may work as supervisors or may teach courses at community colleges. Veterinary technicians might also choose to specialize. While some veterinary technicians eventually become veterinarians, the course of study is not the same, so veterinary technicians cannot simply build on the education they have already received.

SUMMING IT UP

- Veterinary technicians assist veterinarians in providing pets with state-of-the-art veterinary care. A veterinarian technician's duties depend on the size and location of the veterinary practice, but all veterinary technicians provide direct animal care under the supervision of a veterinarian.

- To become a veterinarian technician, you must complete a veterinary technician program accredited by the American Veterinary Medical Association (AVMA). This program leads to a two-year associate degree. Upon graduation, you must pass a comprehensive state examination. Most states give the Veterinary Technician National Examination (VTNE). After this, veterinary technicians apply to be licensed, registered, or certified, depending on the state in which they live.

- Veterinary technicians work in a variety of settings, but the vast majority work in veterinary practices in which the veterinarian specializes in the treatment of small animals such as cats and dogs. Other veterinarians work in large animal practices, animal emergency hospitals, zoos, and biomedical research labs.

- Most states require veterinary assistants to take and pass the Veterinary Technician National Examination (VTNE). This exam contains 225 multiple-choice questions, 200 of which are scored and twenty-five are pilot questions. These questions cover the following subjects, which are also called domains: pharmacy and pharmacology, surgical preparation and assisting, dentistry, laboratory procedures, animal care and nursing, diagnostic imagining, and anesthesia and analgesia.

- While a veterinary technician's salary varies depending on the location and size of the practice, the U.S. Bureau of Labor Statistics reported in 2008 that most veterinary assistants earned an annual salary between $23,580 and $34,960.

- The employment outlook for veterinary assistants is very favorable. The number of veterinary technician jobs is expected to increase 36 percent by 2018. This is much higher than the national average.

- Some veterinary technicians choose to specialize in a particular area or animal. These veterinary technicians must receive certification from an academy, such as the Academy of Veterinary Dental Technicians. Specialization certification usually requires several years' experience as a veterinary technician, additional courses of study, clinical experience, and letters of recommendation. Candidates for specialization are usually also required to take and pass an exam relating to their specialty.

CHAPTER 2

Landing a Job as a Veterinary Technician

OVERVIEW

- **Write your resume**
- **Prepare a cover letter**
- **Browse online job listings**
- **Contact veterinarians in your area**
- **Complete a job application**
- **Prepare for a job interview**
- **Summing it up**

Remember the days when looking for a job consisted of simply scanning the Help Wanted ads in a local newspaper? Do not overlook newspaper classifieds when you begin searching for work as a veterinary technician, but keep in mind that this is only one of many avenues you should take to find a job. If you are especially lucky, you may be offered a job in the veterinary practice where you completed an internship, but this does not always happen. You may have been working in another occupation while pursuing your studies and may have completed a practicum, a long-term project, instead of an internship. And even if you did complete an internship and the veterinarian and his or her staff thought you did a terrific job, they may not have a job opening. In these instances, you need to find a job—and the best way to do this is to search proactively, which means you must take the initiative to find job openings.

WRITE YOUR RESUME

You need to prepare a resume before you start searching for a job. Resume styles vary greatly, but be sure to choose one that is clear and easy to read and that draws attention to your strengths.

Required Sections

Your resume should contain the following sections:

- **Contact Information:** Your contact information includes your name, address, phone number, and e-mail address. If your e-mail address is not professional, get a new one to use during your job search. Many business-people use their first initial and their last name as their e-mail address, as in TSmith@youremailprovider.com.

- **Objective:** Your objective is your goal. The objective of your resume may be as simple as "To obtain a job as a veterinary technician."

- **Education:** List your education on your resume beginning with the most recent. If your resume is short, include a few bulleted points about your course of study. Be sure to include your school's name and address, the dates during which you attended, and the degree you obtained. (See Figure 2-1, "Sample Veterinary Technician Resume.") If your work experience is stronger than your education, list your work experience first. The goal is to make your resume look as impressive as possible.

- **Work Experience:** Begin with the most recent, and keep in mind that it is not necessary to include every job that you have ever held. Include relevant experience, such as experience working with animals or as a receptionist. If you completed an internship, you might want to begin with this. If you held an unrelated job for several years, include this job because it shows that you are reliable.

- **License/Certification/Memberships:** Depending on the state in which you live, indicate that you are licensed or certified. For example, you might add "New Jersey Licensed Animal Health Technician." Also indicate if you belong to any societies, which are also called associations, such as the National Association of Veterinary Technicians in America (NAVTA).

Optional Sections

You might also want to include some of these sections on your resume:

- **References:** Some resumes include two or three references. If you have a reference from a veterinarian or someone who works in a veterinary office, you might want to include this information. Past instructors are also good references. Be sure to ask each individual if it is okay to include him or her as a reference before doing so. It is also fine to write "Available upon Request" after the heading References on your resume.

- **Skills:** Some resumes include a list of skills or special qualifications that look impressive. For example, under the heading "Skills," you might include "Perform laboratory procedures" and "Communicate well with customers."

- **Honors and Awards:** If you have achieved a special honor or award, such as being a member of the National Honor Society in high school, you might want to list this on your resume.

Figure 2-1. Sample Veterinary Technician Resume.

Melanie Harrison
145 Main Street
Apartment D
Philadelphia, PA 19119
(215) 451-0000
MHarrison@youremailprovider.com

OBJECTIVE:
To work in a veterinary practice as a veterinary technician.

SKILLS:
- Provide basic and specialized nursing care
- Obtain and record patient case histories
- Maintain and stock medicine and supplies
- Communicate well with customers
- Collect specimens
- Perform laboratory procedures
- Prepare animals, equipment, and instruments for surgery

EDUCATION:
09-09 to 05-11: Associate's Degree in Veterinary Technology
Central Community College
Philadelphia, PA 19144

EXPERIENCE:
2010–2011: Veterinary Technician Intern
Duties included monitoring medical supplies, providing basic nursing care, monitoring surgical patients, and communicating with veterinarians and clients.
Riverside Veterinary Hospital
715 Main Street
Philadelphia, PA 19119

2008 to present: Shelter Volunteer
Duties included caring for cats and dogs in the shelter; communicating with visitors considering adoption; answering phones; assisting visitors with documentation needed for adoption; communicating with visiting veterinarians.
Skytop Animal Shelter
10 Mountain Terrace
Philadelphia, PA 19119

2005 to 2007: Customer Service Representative (part time)
Duties included answering telephones, taking orders, and entering orders into a database; ensured that orders were shipped on time; frequently communicated with employees in other departments.
Jane's Discount Warehouse
The Mall at Tenth Street
Philadelphia, PA 19119

CERTIFICATION & MEMBERSHIPS:
Pennsylvania Licensed Veterinary Technician
Member of the National Association of Veterinary Technicians in America (NAVTA)
Member of Philadelphia Friends of the Animals

PREPARE A COVER LETTER

You should include a cover letter when you send your resume to veterinary practices and other animal-care facilities. State your purpose in your cover letter, summarize your qualifications, mention any important or interesting information that is not on your resume, and express your interest in working at a particular facility. Your cover letter gives a prospective employer a glimpse of your personality, education, and experience as well as your writing skills. It is not necessary to prepare a different cover letter for every veterinary practice you apply to. Save the body of your letter on a computer and add the date, veterinarian's or office manager's name, and the address of the practice before you send it. Follow these guidelines when writing a cover letter:

- Your name and contact information should be centered at the top of page. Your contact information includes your address, home telephone number, and e-mail address.

- Always include the date flush left.

- Include the name and address of the veterinarian and the practice flush left under the date. You can find the names of veterinarians in your area online or in the phone book. However, if the animal hospital is very large or if you are applying to a shelter, finding the right name might not be so easy. In this case, call ahead and ask who should receive your resume. A large facility might have an office manager or a senior veterinary technician who is in charge of hiring. When sending a cover letter to a veterinarian, always precede his or her name with "Dr."

> **TIP**
>
> Always spell check and carefully proofread your cover letter and resume. Read each of these documents word for word. Put your finger on each word and say it aloud. This will help you spot words that you inadvertently omitted. Have someone else proofread your cover letter and resume as well. Sometimes others will easily spot mistakes that you did not see. A cover letter and resume containing misspelled words and incorrect grammar will not make a good impression on a veterinarian.

- The salutation, or greeting, of your cover letter should simply say, "Dear Dr. [surname]" followed by a colon.

- Take time when drafting the body of your cover letter. Remember that a veterinarian or office manager will form a first impression of you based on your letter. The content of your message may vary, but in general you should do the following:

  - State your name and express your interest in working as a veterinary technician at that particular veterinary practice.

  - Summarize your education and experience. If you do not have relevant experience, include the duties you performed during your internship or skills that you acquired at school.

  - Request an interview and indicate when you are available.

- Close your letter with " Sincerely" followed by a comma. Skip a few spaces and type your name. Sign your name in this space after you print your cover letter.

See Figure 2-2 for a sample cover letter.

Figure 2-2. Your cover letter should be grammatically correct and informative and convey a warm and friendly tone.

Melanie Harrison
145 Main Street
Apartment D
Philadelphia, PA 19119
215-451-0000
MHarrison@youremailprovider.com

January 10, 20--

Dr. Marvin Freeman
Southside Animal Hospital
254 Kennedy Boulevard
Philadelphia, PA 19119

Dear Dr. Freeman:

As a recent graduate of Central Community College with an associate degree in veterinary technology, I am very interested in joining your practice as a veterinary technician.

My education includes an internship at Philadelphia's Riverside Veterinary Hospital, 715 Main Street, under the direction of Dr. Amir Pagani. My duties included conversing with owners to obtain and record patient case histories. Barbara Bennett, a veterinary technician overseeing my training, commended my oral and written communication skills. I also maintained holding areas for animals, provided basic and specialized nursing care, collected specimens, and performed simple laboratory procedures. As a shelter volunteer for several years, I am comfortable working with dogs and cats of all sizes and temperaments. My love of animals is the primary reason that I am pursuing a career as a veterinary technician.

Since no veterinary technician openings are available at Riverside Veterinary Hospital, I am including a copy of a letter of recommendation from Dr. Pagani in which he states that I am well-qualified for an entry-level position as a veterinary technician and would be an asset to any veterinary practice.

I hope you will contact me soon for an interview, even if you do not currently have an opening available. Friends and family have told me that you offer pets exceptional care, and I would really like to meet you and tour your facilities. I hope to be part of your team.

Sincerely,

Melanie Harrison

Melanie Harrison

BROWSE ONLINE JOB LISTINGS

With a click of a mouse, you can find dozens of veterinary technician jobs online. Many search engines allow you to search for these jobs by state. Simply type "Veterinary Technician Jobs in PA," and you will access a listing for job openings in Pennsylvania. If you live in a large city, try searching for jobs within this city. Even your local newspaper most likely posts job ads online.

Also check the Web sites of national societies or associations such as NAVTA. Other associations include the American Veterinary Medical Association (AVMA) and the American Animal Hospital Association (AAHA). Individual states have their own association, which you easily access online.

CONTACT VETERINARIANS IN YOUR AREA

While online listings are helpful in locating a job, some veterinarians do not advertise jobs because they have many resumes on file. This is why it is important to be proactive in your job search. Send your resume and cover letter to veterinarians in your area. You can also drop off your resume and cover letter in person. However, if you do this, make sure you are dressed professionally. (See the "Dress for Success" sidebar in this chapter.) Also be prepared to fill out a job application, even if the veterinarian does not have any openings. You will learn what you need to bring with you to fill out a job application in the next section.

To find a list of veterinarians in your area, access Yellow Pages online or look in the Yellow Pages of your telephone book. Make a list of the veterinary practices in your area. Some of them may have Web sites. If they do, spend a few minutes online to learn about their facilities. You might see something worth mentioning in your cover letter.

Once you have a list, send a cover letter and a resume to each veterinary practice. If your schedule is flexible and you are able to work nights and weekends, send a cover letter and resume to animal emergency clinics, too.

APPLYING FOR JOBS ONLINE

Should you e-mail your resume to prospective employers? If you are responding to a job advertisement that says to apply via e-mail, then you should absolutely e-mail your cover letter and resume. However, when you are contacting veterinarians who are not advertising for a veterinary technician, snail mail is best. Imagine the number of e-mails veterinarians receive in one day. Do you think they replay to—or even read—every e-mail message they receive? Probably not. On the other hand, if you snail mail your resume, the person at the front desk may open it. He or she may be impressed by your qualifications and pass along your resume to the veterinarian or office manager. Furthermore, hardcopy cover letters and resumes are often kept on file while e-mails may be deleted.

COMPLETE A JOB APPLICATION

Most veterinary practices will ask you to complete a job application even if you have submitted a cover letter and a resume. A job application requires you to give specific details about yourself, your education, and your work history. If you are asked to come in for a job interview, expect to complete a job application. You might also be asked to fill out a job application if you are dropping off your cover letter and resume or if you are touring the veterinarian's facilities.

> **TIP**
>
> While it is fine to ask questions after a job interview, refrain from asking about salary, benefits, and time off. It is better to ask questions about the job itself. If you are offered the job, you will be told about salary and other perks.

Gather the following items ahead of time to help you accurately complete a job application:

- Your Social Security card

- Your driver's license

- The name and address of the college you attended and the dates you attended

- A copy of your occupational license, certificate, or registration

- The names, addresses, and phone numbers of your past employers and the dates when you worked there

- The names, phone numbers, and e-mail addresses of three references

While job applications vary, most ask for basically the same information. Reviewing the job application in Figure 2-3 will help you know what to expect.

Figure 2-3. Most job applications ask for very specific information that is not usually included on a resume.

Application for Employment

Personal Employment

Last Name	First	Middle	Date

Street Address	Home Phone ( )-

City, State, Zip

Business Phone ( ) -	E-mail Address:

Are you over 18 years of age? ☐ Yes ☐ No
If not, employment is subject to verification of minimum legal age.

Have you ever applied for employment with us? ☐ Yes ☐ No If Yes: Month and Year _____ Location _____	Social Security No. - -

How did you learn of our organization?

Are you legally eligible for employment in the United States? If no, when will you be able to work?

Are you employed now? If so, may we inquire of your present employer?

Have you ever been convicted of a crime in the past ten years, excluding misdemeanors and summary offenses, which has not been annulled, expunged, or sealed by the court? ☐ Yes ☐ No
If yes, describe in full.

Are there any reasons for which you might not be able to perform the job duties (with a reasonable accommodation)?
☐ Yes ☐ No   If yes, please explain.

Driver's License #	State	Any Violations? ☐ Yes ☐ No

- 1 -

Education

School	Name and location of school	Course of study	No. of years completed	Did you graduate?	Degree or diploma
College				☐ Yes ☐ No	
High				☐ Yes ☐ No	
Trade				☐ Yes ☐ No	
Other				☐ Yes ☐ No	

Military

Complete this section if you served in the U.S. Armed Forces	Branch of Service
Describe your duties and any special training:	Period of Active Duty (Mo. & Yr.) From To
	Rank at Discharge
	Date of Final Discharge

Employment History

Please give accurate, complete full-time and part-time employment record. Start with the present or most recent employer.

	Company Name	Telephone ( ) -
1.	Address	Employed (Start Mo. & Yr.) From To
	Name of Supervisor	Hourly Rate Start Last
	Starting Job Title and Describe Your Work	Reason for Leaving

	Company Name	Telephone ( ) -
2.	Address	Employed (Start Mo. & Yr.) From To
	Name of Supervisor	Hourly Rate Start Last
	Starting Job Title and Describe Your Work	Reason for Leaving
	Company Name	Telephone ( ) -
3.	Address	Employed (Start Mo. & Yr.) From To
	Name of Supervisor	Hourly Rate Start Last
	Starting Job Title and Describe Your Work	Reason for Leaving

We may contact the employers listed above unless you indicate those you do not want us to contact.	Do not contact Employer number(s)_____ Reason_____

References: Below, list the names of three persons not related to you, whom you have known at least one year.

Name	Address	Business	Years Acquainted
1.			
2.			
3.			

The information provided in this Application for Employment is true, correct, and complete. If employed, any misstatements or omissions of fact on this application may result in my dismissal. I understand that acceptance of an offer of employment does not create a contractual obligation upon the employer to continue to employ me in the future.

_____   _____
Date   Signature

PREPARE FOR A JOB INTERVIEW

If a veterinarian has a job opening or anticipates having one in the future, you may be asked to come in for a job interview. A job interview is a chance for a prospective employer to get to know you and determine whether you are a good fit for an organization.

When it comes to job interviews, preparation is the key to success. Always arrive about 10 minutes early for a job interview. If you need to, drive to the veterinarian's office a day or two before the interview so you know exactly where to go and where to park. Gather your clothes and the items you need the night before the interview. Dress casually but professionally. (See the "Dressing for Success" sidebar in this chapter.) Bring a copy of your resume as well as the information and documents you need to complete a job application.

When you arrive at the veterinary practice, be polite and friendly with the staff. Introduce yourself and smile. Understand that veterinary practices are busy places. Be patient and polite with the staff if you are asked to have a seat in the reception area. Respond affectionately to any animals that greet you while you wait. Greet your interviewer with a firm handshake. Do not take a seat until you are told to do so.

Job interviews are stressful. Preparing answers to questions ahead of time and practicing your responses will help you perform well. The following are some common interview questions. Have a friend or family member ask you these and other questions. Always listen to the entire question and wait until the veterinarian has finished speaking to respond. Use correct grammar and avoid using slang in your responses.

- Tell me about yourself. *(Keep in mind that the veterinarian does not want to learn your favorite food. Your response should offer information about your education and work experience. It is also fine to note if you are especially hardworking or a quick learner.)*

- Tell me about the duties you performed during your internship/last job. *(Write out your answer to this question beforehand. While you cannot use your notes during your interview, composing a response will help you provide a good summary of the tasks you completed.)*

- Why do you want to work here? *(It is fine to say that you are eager to begin a career as a veterinary technician, but if you can, think of something specific related to that office. If the staff is warm and friendly and the customers seem happy, mention this.)*

- How do you handle stressful situations? *(Think of some stressful situations in the past. Mention one of these and explain how you coped with the situation. If you were overwhelmed by too many tasks, perhaps you made a to-do list to help you prioritize your work.)*

- Why should I hire you? *(Mention that you are hardworking and eager to learn. Back it up with previous job experience if you can.)*

NOTE

When you interview for a job as a veterinary technician, some of the questions you will be asked will be easy to answer. A veterinarian will likely ask about your education and your experience with customers and animals. Other questions, however, may be more difficult to answer. Some interviewers ask questions such as, "What are your greatest strengths and your greatest weaknesses?" Now, you are probably thinking: *The strength part is easy, but what do I say is my greatest weaknesses?* Choose a weakness that is true, but not serious—and always explain what you have done to overcome this weakness. For example, you might say that your greatest weakness is taking on too much at one time, and you have since learned to ask for help when you need it.

- How would you handle an irate or very upset customer? (*Explain that you would remain calm. Paraphrasing the customer's complaint shows the customer that you understand what he or she is saying. Apologize and inform the customer that you will do everything you can to rectify the situation.*)

Answer the veterinarian's questions honestly and completely. Do not be afraid to say, "No, I don't have experience with that yet, but I would really like to learn." After the interview, thank the veterinarian for his or her time, and follow up with a thank-you note.

Dress for Success

You should dress casually for a job interview at a veterinarian's office—but keep in mind that casual does not mean sloppy. Do not wear jeans, shorts, a t-shirt, sneakers, sandals, or flip-flops. A pair of casual slacks or a casual skirt is best. A button-down shirt is a good option. If you are a woman, wear low-heeled shoes. Make sure your hair is neat and away from your face. Remove any facial piercings. Men should shave all facial hair, although a neatly trimmed beard is often acceptable. Women should wear only light makeup.

SUMMING IT UP

- You need to prepare your resume before you begin looking for a job. A resume lists your contact information, objective, education, employment experience, and licenses/certifications/memberships. Some resumes also include references, special skills that you possess, and honors and awards that you have won.

- You should send a cover letter with your resume. A cover letter states why you are sending your resume, summarizes your education and working experience, and requests an interview.

- Browsing job openings online is one way to search for a job as a veterinary technician. You should also make a list of local veterinarians and mail your resume and cover letter to each of them.

- When you are interviewing for a job, you may be asked to complete a job application. A job application asks for specific information that is usually not included on your resume, such as your Social Security number and the contact information of your former supervisors.

- Preparation is the key to easing your nerves during a job interview. Practice responding to questions that are commonly asked during job interviews.

PART II

Diagnosing Strengths and Weaknesses

ANSWER SHEET PRACTICE TEST 1: DIAGNOSTIC TEST

1. ① ② ③ ④	41. ① ② ③ ④	81. ① ② ③ ④	121. ① ② ③ ④	161. ① ② ③ ④
2. ① ② ③ ④	42. ① ② ③ ④	82. ① ② ③ ④	122. ① ② ③ ④	162. ① ② ③ ④
3. ① ② ③ ④	43. ① ② ③ ④	83. ① ② ③ ④	123. ① ② ③ ④	163. ① ② ③ ④
4. ① ② ③ ④	44. ① ② ③ ④	84. ① ② ③ ④	124. ① ② ③ ④	164. ① ② ③ ④
5. ① ② ③ ④	45. ① ② ③ ④	85. ① ② ③ ④	125. ① ② ③ ④	165. ① ② ③ ④
6. ① ② ③ ④	46. ① ② ③ ④	86. ① ② ③ ④	126. ① ② ③ ④	166. ① ② ③ ④
7. ① ② ③ ④	47. ① ② ③ ④	87. ① ② ③ ④	127. ① ② ③ ④	167. ① ② ③ ④
8. ① ② ③ ④	48. ① ② ③ ④	88. ① ② ③ ④	128. ① ② ③ ④	168. ① ② ③ ④
9. ① ② ③ ④	49. ① ② ③ ④	89. ① ② ③ ④	129. ① ② ③ ④	169. ① ② ③ ④
10. ① ② ③ ④	50. ① ② ③ ④	90. ① ② ③ ④	130. ① ② ③ ④	170. ① ② ③ ④
11. ① ② ③ ④	51. ① ② ③ ④	91. ① ② ③ ④	131. ① ② ③ ④	171. ① ② ③ ④
12. ① ② ③ ④	52. ① ② ③ ④	92. ① ② ③ ④	132. ① ② ③ ④	172. ① ② ③ ④
13. ① ② ③ ④	53. ① ② ③ ④	93. ① ② ③ ④	133. ① ② ③ ④	173. ① ② ③ ④
14. ① ② ③ ④	54. ① ② ③ ④	94. ① ② ③ ④	134. ① ② ③ ④	174. ① ② ③ ④
15. ① ② ③ ④	55. ① ② ③ ④	95. ① ② ③ ④	135. ① ② ③ ④	175. ① ② ③ ④
16. ① ② ③ ④	56. ① ② ③ ④	96. ① ② ③ ④	136. ① ② ③ ④	176. ① ② ③ ④
17. ① ② ③ ④	57. ① ② ③ ④	97. ① ② ③ ④	137. ① ② ③ ④	177. ① ② ③ ④
18. ① ② ③ ④	58. ① ② ③ ④	98. ① ② ③ ④	138. ① ② ③ ④	178. ① ② ③ ④
19. ① ② ③ ④	59. ① ② ③ ④	99. ① ② ③ ④	139. ① ② ③ ④	179. ① ② ③ ④
20. ① ② ③ ④	60. ① ② ③ ④	100. ① ② ③ ④	140. ① ② ③ ④	180. ① ② ③ ④
21. ① ② ③ ④	61. ① ② ③ ④	101. ① ② ③ ④	141. ① ② ③ ④	181. ① ② ③ ④
22. ① ② ③ ④	62. ① ② ③ ④	102. ① ② ③ ④	142. ① ② ③ ④	182. ① ② ③ ④
23. ① ② ③ ④	63. ① ② ③ ④	103. ① ② ③ ④	143. ① ② ③ ④	183. ① ② ③ ④
24. ① ② ③ ④	64. ① ② ③ ④	104. ① ② ③ ④	144. ① ② ③ ④	184. ① ② ③ ④
25. ① ② ③ ④	65. ① ② ③ ④	105. ① ② ③ ④	145. ① ② ③ ④	185. ① ② ③ ④
26. ① ② ③ ④	66. ① ② ③ ④	106. ① ② ③ ④	146. ① ② ③ ④	186. ① ② ③ ④
27. ① ② ③ ④	67. ① ② ③ ④	107. ① ② ③ ④	147. ① ② ③ ④	187. ① ② ③ ④
28. ① ② ③ ④	68. ① ② ③ ④	108. ① ② ③ ④	148. ① ② ③ ④	188. ① ② ③ ④
29. ① ② ③ ④	69. ① ② ③ ④	109. ① ② ③ ④	149. ① ② ③ ④	189. ① ② ③ ④
30. ① ② ③ ④	70. ① ② ③ ④	110. ① ② ③ ④	150. ① ② ③ ④	190. ① ② ③ ④
31. ① ② ③ ④	71. ① ② ③ ④	111. ① ② ③ ④	151. ① ② ③ ④	191. ① ② ③ ④
32. ① ② ③ ④	72. ① ② ③ ④	112. ① ② ③ ④	152. ① ② ③ ④	192. ① ② ③ ④
33. ① ② ③ ④	73. ① ② ③ ④	113. ① ② ③ ④	153. ① ② ③ ④	193. ① ② ③ ④
34. ① ② ③ ④	74. ① ② ③ ④	114. ① ② ③ ④	154. ① ② ③ ④	194. ① ② ③ ④
35. ① ② ③ ④	75. ① ② ③ ④	115. ① ② ③ ④	155. ① ② ③ ④	195. ① ② ③ ④
36. ① ② ③ ④	76. ① ② ③ ④	116. ① ② ③ ④	156. ① ② ③ ④	196. ① ② ③ ④
37. ① ② ③ ④	77. ① ② ③ ④	117. ① ② ③ ④	157. ① ② ③ ④	197. ① ② ③ ④
38. ① ② ③ ④	78. ① ② ③ ④	118. ① ② ③ ④	158. ① ② ③ ④	198. ① ② ③ ④
39. ① ② ③ ④	79. ① ② ③ ④	119. ① ② ③ ④	159. ① ② ③ ④	199. ① ② ③ ④
40. ① ② ③ ④	80. ① ② ③ ④	120. ① ② ③ ④	160. ① ② ③ ④	200. ① ② ③ ④

CHAPTER 3

Practice Test 1— Diagnostic Test

1. All the following inhaled anesthetic drugs should be used with a rebreathing system *except*:
   1. halothane.
   2. isoflurane.
   3. nitrous oxide.
   4. desflurane.

2. You should bury the needle in the vein of which of the following animals when taking a blood sample?
   1. Persian cat
   2. Golden retriever
   3. Oriental cat
   4. Pomeranian

3. Which of the following would contraindicate the administration of morphine as a preanesthetic agent?
   1. Preexisting tachycardia
   2. Liver disease
   3. Gastrointestinal obstruction
   4. Respiratory disease

4. All the following pieces of information would be subject to the confidentiality requirements of patients' medical records *except a*:
   1. report of injuries sustained as a result of abuse.
   2. report of a contagious or zoonotic disease.
   3. record of a patient's vaccination history.
   4. record of abnormal behavioral.

5. An abscess is best described as a/an:
   1. abnormal communication between the oral and nasal cavities.
   2. collection of material from a bacterial infection in the tooth.
   3. tooth that can't break past the gum surface.
   4. hole or chip in the tooth.

6. Which medication would be given to a patient experiencing constipation?
   1. Oxazepam
   2. Ranitidine
   3. Bisacodyl
   4. Apomorphine

7. A cholinergic is a drug that:
   1. decreases pain sensations.
   2. blocks the action of adrenaline at beta-adrenergic receptors.
   3. causes pupil dilation.
   4. stimulates the parasympathetic nervous system.

8. When disposing of a used needle, you should:
   1. destroy the needle and dispose of it in the appropriate container.
   2. separate the needle and syringe and dispose of it in the appropriate container.
   3. recap the needle and dispose of it in the appropriate container.
   4. handle the needle carefully and dispose of it in the appropriate container.

9. You are treating a dehydrated dog that presents with sunken eyes, increased CRT, and dry mucus membranes. What is the patient's estimated degree of dehydration?
   1. 5–6% dehydration
   2. 8% dehydration
   3. 10–12% dehydration
   4. 12–15% dehydration

10. A veterinary technician receives a frantic call from a pet owner. From what the owner says, the technician concludes the owner's dog is experiencing gastric dilation and volvulus. In which of the following categories of emergency should the technician place the patient?
    1. Nonemergency
    2. Minor
    3. Serious
    4. Life threatening

11. Barium is considered a/an:
    1. soluble positive contrast medium.
    2. insoluble negative contrast medium.
    3. soluble negative contrast medium.
    4. insoluble positive contrast medium.

12. Trichiasis *most* commonly affects which breed of canine?
    1. English bulldog
    2. Poodle
    3. Pug
    4. Cocker spaniel

13. A surgeon uses Jacobs chucks to:
    1. break up and remove bone.
    2. hold bone fragments in reduction.
    3. cut through bone.
    4. advance pin placement.

14. Which of the following would be considered a poor inventory control practice?
    1. Using control cards or a computer system for inventory control
    2. Closely monitoring expiration dates of the stored products
    3. Purchasing the most affordable medications possible
    4. Arranging medications based on frequency of use

15. Which of the following drugs would be used to reduce intracranial pressure?
    1. Atropine
    2. Pimobendan
    3. Mannitol
    4. Prazosin

16. Which of the following statements would be true of the anesthetic agent guaifenesin?
    1. It crosses the placental barrier but has no effect on the fetus.
    2. It crosses the placental barrier but has little effect on the fetus.
    3. It doesn't cross the placental barrier and has no effect on the fetus.
    4. It doesn't cross the placental barrier and has little effect on the fetus.

17. A healthy horse should have a white blood cell count ranging from:
    1. 3–10.
    2. 6–12.
    3. 6–17.
    4. 7–14.

18. Which of the following should be used to detect external odontoclastic resorptive lesions in a cat?
    1. Periodontal probe
    2. Shepherd's hook
    3. Curette
    4. Sickle scaler

19. Which physical factor might result in diminished radiographic detail in an X-ray?
    1. Ineffective filtration
    2. Low subject contrast
    3. Patient movement
    4. Negative contrast use

20. Canine patients should be placed in lateral recumbency when extracting a blood sample from which vein?
    1. Jugular vein
    2. Cephalic vein
    3. Saphenous vein
    4. Femoral vein

21. When preparing a patient for a blood sample collection from the cephalic vein, the restrainer should:
    1. hold the patient's front legs with one hand and its head with the other while extending the neck.
    2. place the fingers of one hand behind the patient's elbow to extend the front leg.
    3. hold the patient's distal thigh or proximal tibia to compress the vein while extending the stifle.
    4. compress the vein by placing one hand on the medial side of the upper thigh.

22. Which cardiovascular drug serves to provide long-term maintenance of contractibility?
    1. Dobutamine
    2. Hydralazine
    3. Propranolol
    4. Digoxin

23. Tissue forceps with multiple fine, intermeshing teeth on the edges are known as:
    1. Brown-Adson tissue forceps.
    2. Rat-tooth thumb forceps.
    3. Adson tissue forceps.
    4. Russian tissue forceps.

24. A feline blood donor *must* weigh no less than:
    1. 5 pounds.
    2. 8 pounds.
    3. 10 pounds.
    4. 12 pounds.

25. You are treating a dog with itchy patches around the ears, chest, abdomen, and front legs. Which of the following is *most likely* to be the correct diagnosis?
    1. Demodectic mange
    2. Walking dandruff
    3. Sarcoptic mange
    4. Fleas

26. You are experiencing a conflict with a colleague. Which of the following approaches to the situation would be *least likely* to lead to a positive outcome?
    1. Have a face-to-face conversation.
    2. Bring up the issue at a staff meeting.
    3. File a formal, written complaint.
    4. Allow the problem to resolve itself.

27. Azaperone is *most* often used as a preanesthetic for:
    1. pigs.
    2. dogs.
    3. cats.
    4. birds.

28. When developing an X-ray, what is the primary purpose of the rinse bath?
    1. To begin the development process on the film
    2. To convert the exposed silver halide crystals to metallic silver
    3. To clear away the underexposed silver halide crystals
    4. To stop the process of development and prevent contamination of the fixer

29. Which anesthetic agent would be *most* appropriate for use with a greyhound?
    1. Etomidate
    2. Cyclohexamine
    3. Propofol
    4. Fentanyl

30. How much hair should be removed from either side of the midline in a large dog being prepared for surgery?
    1. 2 inches
    2. 3 inches
    3. 4 inches
    4. 5 inches

31. Which term refers to the tooth surface area that faces towards the cheek?
    1. Buccal
    2. Labial
    3. Rostral
    4. Occlusal

32. When protected with wrapping material and kept on an open shelf, up to how long can a surgical instrument remain sterile?
    1. One week
    2. Two weeks
    3. Three weeks
    4. Four weeks

33. Which of the following would be a normal sulcus depth for a cat?
    1. Less than 0.5 millimeters
    2. Less than 1 millimeter
    3. More than 1 millimeter
    4. More than 1.5 millimeters

34. Which of the following would be a sign of overhydration?
    1. Lowered blood pressure
    2. Decreased lung sounds
    3. Fatigue
    4. Chemosis

35. Which substance commonly used in wound lavage may result in tissue damage?
1. Isotonic saline
2. Hydrogen peroxide
3. Chlorhexidine diacetate solution
4. Povidone-iodine solution

36. A veterinary technician has a question about whether a certain practice is ethical. Which of the following resources would be the best place to find answers to an ethical problem in the veterinary workplace?
1. The technician's own sense of morality and ethics
2. The technician's state laws and codes about veterinary medicine
3. A veterinary medicine professional organization
4. A friend of the technician who doesn't work in veterinary medicine

37. Which of the following is the *most commonly* used anticoagulant for blood testing?
1. Oxalate
2. Heparin
3. EDTA
4. Sodium citrate

38. Which of the following drugs is used as an immunosuppressant agent?
1. Dextran
2. Lactulose
3. Interferon
4. Auranofin

39. On an X-ray, denser body parts will appear:
1. darker.
2. whiter.
3. grayer.
4. foggier.

40. Which of the following dog breeds is at a higher risk for hip dysplasia?
1. Chihuahua
2. Mastiff
3. Jack Russell terrier
4. Greyhound

41. In order to achieve the *most* accurate diagnosis, an X-ray should always be taken from at least how many angles?
1. One
2. Two
3. Three
4. Four

42. Which of the following barbiturates has a lethal dosage only two to three times its normal anesthetic dosage?
1. Thiopental
2. Pentobarbital
3. Methohexital
4. Phenobarbital

43. When using a non-rebreathing system during anesthesia, the fresh gas flow rate should be set between:
1. 85 to 115 mL/kg/min.
2. 100 to 130 mL/kg/min.
3. 130 to 300 mL/kg/min.
4. 300 to 400 mL/kg/min.

44. Which of the following is a synthetic absorbable suture material?
1. Polydioxanone
2. Polypropylene
3. Polyamide
4. Polymerized caprolactam

45. A dog presents with a dental malocclusion in which two of the maxillary incisors are displaced so that they are lingual to the mandibular incisors. This condition is referred to as:
1. posterior crossbite.
2. anterior crossbite.
3. distocclusion.
4. mesiocclusion.

46. Which of the following species develops only one set of teeth during its lifetime?
1. Horse
2. Sheep
3. Rabbit
4. Swine

47. A medication delivered intraosseously is injected into:
    1. the skin.
    2. the bone cavity.
    3. a muscle.
    4. a blood vessel.

48. Veterinary technicians are sometimes the first people in a veterinary office to see a patient. As this is a major responsibility, they must be able to categorize the patient into the appropriate emergency group. An example of a patient with a serious emergency would be a:
    1. dog with a bee sting.
    2. cat with a minor burn.
    3. bird with a gaping wound.
    4. ferret with an abscess.

49. Which of the following should a veterinary technician do in case of an accidental perivascular administration of diazepam?
    1. Rapidly inject sterile saline into the injection site.
    2. Slowly inject sterile saline into the injection site.
    3. Rapidly inject lidocaine to numb the injection site.
    4. Slowly inject lidocaine to numb the injection site.

50. Catgut, a commonly used absorbable suture material, is made from the submucosal layer of the intestines of which animal?
    1. Cats
    2. Sheep
    3. Dogs
    4. Cattle

51. Which of the following antimicrobial drug types functions by interfering with DNA/RNA synthesis?
    1. Penicillin
    2. Ketoconazole
    3. Tetracycline
    4. Amoxicillin

52. Which of the following drugs is a nonsteroidal anti-inflammatory drug (NSAID)?
    1. Betamethasone
    2. Hyaluronate
    3. Methocarbamol
    4. Etodolac

53. Which of the following X-ray processing errors would result in a yellow radiograph?
    1. Marks left by fingerprints
    2. Exhausted fixer solution
    3. Low developing solution
    4. High drying temperature

54. Which top color indicates a Vacutainer containing only EDTA and no other additives?
    1. Red
    2. Lavender
    3. Light blue
    4. Dark blue

55. The use of which type of anesthetic agent would be contraindicated in a patient with glaucoma?
    1. Etomidate
    2. Cyclohexamine
    2. Fentanyl
    3. Propofol

56. Which inhaled anesthetic is best suited for avian species?
    1. Sevoflurane
    2. Desflurane
    3. Isoflurane
    4. Halothane

57. A lower grid ratio would indicate that:
    1. less scatter radiation is absorbed.
    2. more scatter radiation is absorbed.
    3. more primary radiation is being emitted.
    4. less primary radiation is being emitted.

58. Which of the following is classified as a colloid?
    1. Hartmann's solution
    2. Lactated Ringer's solution
    3. Pentastarch
    4. Saline

59. Which of the following is a canine blood parasite?
    1. Ehrlichia canis
    2. Babesia canis
    3. Ehrlichia platys
    4. Borrelia burgdorferi

60. Finochietto retractors are commonly used during what type of surgery?
1. Abdominal
2. Neurosurgery
3. Orthopedic
4. Thoracic

61. Which of the following is described as a loss of radiographic detail common with faster screens because of unevenly distributed phosphor crystals within the intensifying screen?
1. Penumbra
2. Quantum mottle
3. Structure mottle
4. Radiographic mottle

62. When taking a small volume blood sample from a cow, the blood is *most frequently* extracted from the:
1. milk vein.
2. jugular vein.
3. caudal auricular vein.
4. tail vein.

63. Which type of imaging test involves injecting dye into the spinal canal in order to highlight small changes in the spinal cord?
1. Nuclear scintigraphy
2. Myelography
3. MRI
4. Endoscopy

64. Which canine species is *most* commonly associated with gingival hyperplasia?
1. Pug
2. Scottish terrier
3. Boxer
4. Dachshund

65. The *most* common type of oral tumor among dogs is:
1. fibrosarcoma.
2. melanoma.
3. osteosarcoma.
4. squamous cell carcinoma.

66. A cat with type AB blood may receive:
1. type A blood.
2. type B blood.
3. type AB blood.
4. any feline blood type.

67. Which anesthetic agent may result in an increase in cerebrospinal fluid pressure?
1. Halothane
2. Guaifenesin
3. Isoflurane
4. Sevoflurane

68. Which size needle is most commonly used for venipuncture in cats and small dogs?
1. 18 gauge
2. 20 gauge
3. 22 gauge
4. 24 gauge

69. You are treating a cat that has consumed a non-caustic toxin. Which of the following drugs would you administer in order to induce vomiting?
1. Chlorpromazine
2. Xylazine
3. Metoclopramide
4. Aminopentamide

70. After a surgery on a dog, you are asked to disinfect. On which surface could you safely use bleach to disinfect?
1. The dog's skin and wounds
2. The metal operating table
3. The steel surgical instruments
4. The linoleum floors

71. Which of the following antiemetic drugs would be prescribed for an animal experiencing chemotherapy sickness?
1. Dimenhydrinate
2. Meclizine
3. Metoclopramide
4. Ondansetron

72. Which type of chew toy can lead to gingival trauma?
1. Nylon rope toys
2. Dried hooves
3. Nylon chew bones
4. Rawhide strips

73. Radiographic detail can be increased by:
1. increasing the source-image distance.
2. decreasing the source-image distance.
3. increasing the object-film distance.
4. increasing the kVp level.

74. Which of the following is the definitive means of diagnosing a malignant tumor?
    1. Cytology
    2. Radiography
    3. Histopathology
    4. Serum chemistry profile

75. Which of the following is a negative effect of an improperly applied bandage?
    1. Wound drainage
    2. Immobilization of a limb
    3. Tissue necrosis
    4. Wound debridement

76. The minimum weight for a canine blood donor is:
    1. 25 pounds.
    2. 45 pounds.
    3. 55 pounds.
    4. 65 pounds.

77. Which of the following species requires sedation or anesthesia for venipuncture?
    1. Mongolian gerbil
    2. Mouse
    3. Rat
    4. Guinea pig

78. All the following antimicrobial medications can be administered to rabbits *except*:
    1. clindamycin.
    2. lincomycin.
    3. erythromycin.
    4. tylosin.

79. During a surgical procedure, a canine patient develops malignant hyperthermia. With what drug should the patient be treated?
    1. Calcium EDTA
    2. Dantrolene
    3. Pamidronate
    4. Atropine

80. In an induction that does *not* go smoothly, which normally bypassed stage is experienced?
    1. Stage 1
    2. Stage 2
    3. Stage 3
    4. Stage 4

81. When using a Bard-Parker scalpel handle during a small animal surgical procedure, which blade would you use with a Number 3 handle to sever ligaments?
    1. Number 10
    2. Number 11
    3. Number 12
    4. Number 15

82. A high dose of which of the following preanesthetic agents could be dangerous for a ruminant?
    1. Droperidol
    2. Xylazine
    3. Azaperone
    4. Acepromazine

83. An excessively high level of what vitamin is thought to be a possible contributing factor in the development of feline odontoclastic resorptive lesions?
    1. Vitamin A
    2. Vitamin B_{12}
    3. Vitamin C
    4. Vitamin D

84. Veterinary technicians sometimes use tourniquets to immobilize limbs and stop blood. The recommended maximum amount of time a tourniquet should be used is:
    1. 5 minutes.
    2. 20 minutes.
    3. 40 minutes.
    4. 60 minutes.

85. Which teeth are absent in lagomorphs?
    1. Incisors
    2. Canines
    3. Premolars
    4. Molars

86. In guinea pigs, what dental condition is associated with vitamin C deficiency?
    1. Malocclusion
    2. Caries
    3. Overgrowth
    4. Periodontal disease

87. An accurate statement concerning slow speed screens would be that they:
    1. produce average quality resolution radiographs with relatively low exposures.
    2. are used when increased patient penetration is needed.
    3. are designed to produce optimum detail with little regard to exposure time.
    4. normally have a thicker phosphor layer.

88. Which of the following is a cause of sinus bradycardia?
    1. Hyperthyroidism
    2. Anemia
    3. Increased cerebrospinal fluid pressure
    4. Reduced cardiac output

89. Manual compression of the bladder would be an appropriate method for:
    1. examining solute concentration in urine.
    2. relieving bladder distention due to obstruction.
    3. collecting a sterile urine sample for urinalysis and culture.
    4. clearing a urethral obstruction.

90. Halsted mosquito forceps have:
    1. distal transverse grooves.
    2. transverse serrations covering the entire jaw length.
    3. complete transverse grooves.
    4. longitudinal grooves and distal transverse grooves.

91. When cutting and dissecting dense tissue, a veterinary surgeon would *most likely* use:
    1. Metzenbaum scissors.
    2. Iris scissors.
    3. Spencer scissors.
    4. Mayo scissors.

92. Miconazole is used to treat:
    1. gastrointestinal and skin *Candida* infections.
    2. dermatophytosis or avian mycoses.
    3. fungal ophthalmic infections.
    4. inflammatory bowel disease.

93. Which inhaled anesthetic has the highest rate of metabolization?
    1. Halothane
    2. Sevoflurane
    3. Nitrous oxide
    4. Desflurane

94. When collecting a blood sample that should clot, you should use a Vacutainer with which color top?
    1. Green
    2. Blue
    3. Red
    4. Black

95. Which type of anesthetic agent is most useful for patients with cardiac disease?
    1. Cyclohexamines
    2. Barbiturates
    3. Propofol
    4. Etomidate

96. The reduction of orally administered drugs in the liver is known as:
    1. perfusion.
    2. first-pass effect.
    3. diffusion.
    4. second-pass metabolism.

97. During a venipuncture, when the needle is removed from the vein, you should immediately:
    1. place the sample into a Vacutainer.
    2. stop compression of the vein.
    3. apply pressure over the venipuncture site.
    4. release the patient from restraint.

98. According to the American Society of Anesthesiologists scale, a patient with fever, anemia, heart murmur, and moderate dehydration would be considered a:
    1. Category II patient.
    2. Category III patient.
    3. Category IV patient.
    4. Category V patient.

99. Which of the following best describes the meaning of *uveitis*?
    1. Decreased tear production and corneal film
    2. Inflammation of the eye's middle vascular layer
    3. Corneal inflammation
    4. Squinting or crossing of the eyes

100. When performing a surgical scrub, you should begin at the:
1. incision and work outward in a circular motion.
2. fringes of the surgical area and work inward in a circular motion
3. incision and work outward in a back-and-forth motion.
4. fringes of the surgical area and work inward in a back-and-forth motion.

101. A woman finds her dog drinking drain cleaner and immediately brings it to the veterinary clinic. Which of the following treatments would be *most* appropriate in this scenario?
1. Administer an emetic
2. Administer activated charcoal
3. Administer kaolin
4. Administer milk and monitor

102. How long must a dog that has just been vaccinated wait before donating blood?
1. Two weeks
2. Five days
3. One week
4. Twelve days

103. Newborn animals must be kept in warm facilities up to four weeks after birth. During the first ten days, how warm should the temperature of the room be?
1. 55–60°F
2. 65–70°F
3. 75–80°F
4. 85–90°F

104. Distichiasis results in:
1. a second row of eyelashes.
2. ingrown eyelash hairs.
3. glandular tissue that projects beyond the haw.
4. squinting or crossing of the eyes.

105. Which of the following would be described as a self-retaining forceps commonly used for holding bowels?
1. Allis tissue forceps
2. Babcock intestinal forceps
3. Doyen intestinal forceps
4. Ferguson angiotribe forceps

106. Which of the following techniques would contribute to a successful venipuncture attempt?
1. Inserting the needle downward toward the patient
2. Retracting the syringe plunger as quickly as possible
3. Inserting the needle upward toward the ceiling
4. Fully retracting the syringe plunger immediately upon puncture

107. Which anesthetic agent is dangerous to use on horses and cattle?
1. Fentanyl
2. Propofol
3. Guaifenesin
4. Etomidate

108. When packing a biopsy sample for shipping, you should:
1. ensure the sample remains completely dry during shipping.
2. freeze the sample and put it on dry ice to keep it cold for shipping.
3. add an appropriate fluid to the container to soak the sample.
4. heat the sample and separate it from cold samples during shipping.

109. Use of which inhaled anesthetic will result in a lessened or absent version of the hangover effect that normally accompanies inhaled anesthetics?
1. Sevoflurane
2. Desflurane
3. Isoflurane
4. Halothane

110. A drug with a high therapeutic index has:
1. a high toxicity level.
2. a low toxicity level.
3. numerous side effects.
4. numerous benefits.

111. Which adrenergic agent is used to treat urinary incontinence?
1. Dopamine
2. Terbutaline
3. Phenylpropanolamine
4. Epinephrine

112. You suspect a patient at your clinic has been poisoned by antifreeze. Which of the following samples should you collect to test for antifreeze?
    1. Blood
    2. Serum
    3. Urine
    4. Hair

113. What canine breed is predisposed to seborrhea oleosa?
    1. German shepherd
    2. Pug
    3. Dalmatian
    4. Cocker spaniel

114. If a sterile item touches a nonsterile item, it should be:
    1. quickly sterilized for immediate use.
    2. immediately discarded.
    3. rinsed with soap and water and reused.
    4. placed on a nonsterile tray.

115. Which of the following methods would be used to monitor the oxygenation of a patient under anesthesia?
    1. Auscultation of breath sounds
    2. Observing the chest wall
    3. Observing mucus membrane color
    4. Capnography

116. Which canine breed is often sensitive to the cardiovascular drug digoxin?
    1. Great Dane
    2. Golden retriever
    3. Irish setter
    4. Doberman pinscher

117. You've just collected a urine sample that you will send to a laboratory for testing. Which of the following actions would you *most likely* take with the sample?
    1. Dilute it
    2. Heat it
    3. Centrifuge it
    4. Freeze it

118. What surgical instrument is sometimes used to scrape out osteochondritis dissecans lesions?
    1. Osteotome
    2. Bone curette
    3. Bone rasp
    4. Rongeur

119. Before giving a patient anesthesia, veterinary technicians go through multiple stages of procedures to ensure the patient's health and safety. All these actions are taken when the technician is assessing the patient's medical history *except*:
    1. asking if the patient's vaccinations are updated.
    2. determining the status of the patient's overall health.
    3. asking about adverse reactions to drugs.
    4. determining the patient's vital signs.

120. You collected laboratory specimens from a patient who has been on a high-protein diet. The patient's laboratory test results will *most likely* show the patient's:
    1. urea nitrogen levels have increased.
    2. bile concentrations have increased.
    3. acid concentrations have increased.
    4. ALT levels have increased.

121. Which inhaled anesthetic requires an agent specific out-of-circle precision vaporizer?
    1. Desflurane
    2. Isoflurane
    3. Halothane
    4. Sevoflurane

122. Which veterinary surgical procedure requires no hair removal during patient preparation?
    1. Feline castration
    2. Perineal urethrostomy
    3. Canine castration
    4. Laparotomy

123. A centrifuge's speed is measured in:
    1. d forces.
    2. e forces.
    3. g forces.
    4. p forces.

124. Opioid analgesics relieve pain by:
    1. reducing inflammation.
    2. blocking the brain's pain impulses.
    3. producing local anesthesia.
    4. blocking prostaglandin production.

125. Operating room personnel who have been chronically exposed to nitrous oxide may be at increased risk of what condition?
    1. Hepatotoxicity
    2. Renal dysfunction
    3. Liver damage
    4. Myeloneuropathy

126. Which method of euthanasia is performed only on very small animals?
    1. Intracardiac injection
    2. Enclosed chamber
    3. Intravenous injection
    4. Intraperitoneal injection

127. Which of the following best describes the technique of fanning during an ultrasound?
    1. Keeping the transducer in one place and applying pressure to the front or the back
    2. Holding the transducer in one place and titling it from side to side
    3. Holding the transducer in an upright position and moving in different directions
    4. Keeping the transducer in contact with skin while pivoting it 90°

128. If a patient suffers from spinal dysfunctions, the first step in diagnosing the problem is *most likely*:
    1. the collection of a blood sample.
    2. a radiography screening.
    3. the collection of a stool sample.
    4. a surgical biopsy.

129. A dog is excited and panting before a radiography screening. Your team might consider giving the dog a light sedative because the dog's panting:
    1. could fog the screen, making it difficult to see the results.
    2. may annoy members of the veterinary team.
    3. may move the animal's body and compromise the results.
    4. could be loud and distracting to the radiographer.

130. Anesthetics are used for a variety of reasons in veterinary medicine. Radiographers *most likely* use anesthetics for:
    1. anesthesia.
    2. euthanasia.
    3. restraint.
    4. seizure control.

131. Small amounts of white light have come in contact with radiographic images in the darkroom. The images will *most likely* become:
    1. completely black.
    2. slightly foggy.
    3. completely white.
    4. slightly clearer.

132. In which of the following positions is an animal lying on its back?
    1. Dorsal recumbency
    2. Right lateral recumbency
    3. Left lateral recumbency
    4. Sternal recumbency

133. Which of the following opioids is *most* potent?
    1. Buprenorphine
    2. Meperidine
    3. Morphine
    4. Fentanyl

134. Which form of sterilization is the preferred method for instruments that are used during surgery?
    1. Autoclaving
    2. Chemical sterilization
    3. Boiling
    4. Dry heat

135. When preparing a bovine's skin for surgery, which of the following steps should be completed first?
    1. Clip most of the fur from the skin.
    2. Disinfect the skin with an iodine solution.
    3. Wash the skin with soap and water.
    4. Disinfect the skin with an alcohol solution.

136. For which of the following procedures is epidural anesthesia *most* effective?
    1. Cataract surgery
    2. Tooth extraction
    3. Throat surgery
    4. Tail amputation

137. Which of the following is *not* a disorder that causes coagulation problems for animals?
    1. Hemophilia
    2. Liver disease
    3. Vitamin K deficiency
    4. Vitamin A deficiency

138. On average, at what percentage of blood loss do small animals (e.g., cats and dogs) begin to experience symptoms of acute blood loss?
1. 5–10%
2. 15–20%
3. 35–40%
4. 45–50%

139. You are collecting blood samples from a patient using an EDTA tube. If you fill the EDTA tube with too little blood you could alter the test results because the:
1. sample could have a decreased packed cell volume.
2. EDTA could cause poorly stained leukocytes.
3. sample could show a false increase in sodium levels.
4. EDTA could make bile measurements unreliable.

140. Which ophthalmic drug would be used to constrict the pupil?
1. Tetracaine
2. Atropine
3. Cyclosporine
4. Pilocarpine

141. Which diuretic can be administered intramuscularly?
1. Furosemide
2. Spironolactone
3. Chlorothiazide
4. Mannitol

142. When checking a high-pressure anesthetic machine for leaks, you would be *most likely* to find a leak in the:
1. unidirectional valves.
2. tank yoke connectors.
3. pop-off valve.
4. soda lime canister.

143. Prostaglandins are administered to:
1. prevent pregnancy after mismating.
2. lyse the corpus luteum.
3. return a mare in transitional anestrus to proestrus.
4. induce uterine contractions.

144. The Bain system breathing circuit is most useful with patients undergoing procedures involving what part of the body?
1. Legs
2. Chest
3. Head
4. Spine

145. Which inhaled anesthetic is no longer commonly used because of its potential severe side effects?
1. Sevoflurane
2. Halothane
3. Isoflurane
4. Methoxyflurane

146. Which antiparasitic drug *cannot* be administered to cats because of potential toxicity?
1. Selamectin
2. Amitraz
3. Imidacloprid
4. Nitenpyram

147. Which of the following is true of non-precision vaporizers?
1. They make anesthesia depth difficult to control.
2. They compensate for temperature and back-pressure.
3. They are generally very expensive.
4. They must be serviced every six to twelve months.

148. Nitrous oxide is:
1. a nonflammable, non-explosive halogenated ether.
2. highly pungent and irritative to the airway.
3. highly reactive to metals.
4. nonirritative and sweet smelling.

149. Dimercaprol can be used to treat a patient suffering from:
1. poisonous snake envenomation.
2. opioid agonist reversal.
3. mercury toxicity.
4. serotonin syndrome.

150. Which type of barbiturate is most often used as a sedative for excitable dogs?
1. Pentobarbital
2. Phenobarbital
3. Methohexital
4. Thiopental

151. An adult female dog shows signs of pseudocyesis. With which medication would the patient *most likely* be treated?
1. Oxytocin
2. Mibolerone
3. Desmopressin
4. Medroxy-progesterone

152. Which of the following is true about etomidate?
1. It supports bacterial growth due to soy content.
2. It is reconstituted with water or dextrose.
3. It is referred to as a neuroleptanalgesic.
4. It may cause phlebitis upon injection.

153. Which antifungal medication is known to cause birth defects or spontaneous abortion in cats?
1. Nystatin
2. Fluconazole
3. Griseofulvin
4. Terbinafine

154. After surgery, the medical team has a certain amount of time to clean and close an open wound. How much time can elapse before the cleaning and closing of a wound before a wound is likely to become infected?
1. 10 to 20 minutes
2. 40 to 50 minutes
3. 1 to 2 hours
4. 4 to 6 hours

155. Which nonabsorbable suture material may act like a wick and allow the migration of contamination?
1. Polypropylene
2. Stainless steel
3. Nylon
4. Silk

156. Anesthetization with which inhalant should be avoided in patients with respiratory problems that affect their ability to oxygenate?
1. Halothane
2. Nitrous oxide
3. Sevoflurane
4. Isoflurane

157. H2 blockers are systemic antacids designed to:
1. prevent the production of hydrochloric acid.
2. block the release of hydrogen ions and stimulate mucus.
3. prevent the pumping of hydrogen ions into the stomach.
4. neutralize acid that is already present in the stomach.

158. One sign of infection in a patient is inflammation. All of these are symptoms of inflammation *except*:
1. Loss of function
2. Swelling
3. Presence of puss
4. Redness

159. Which of the following cardiovascular drugs is a calcium channel blocker?
1. Isoproterenol
2. Pimobendan
3. Diltiazem
4. Captopril

160. When clipping an animal for surgery on an open wound, you should place water-soluble lubricant in the wound in order to:
1. decontaminate the wound.
2. encourage faster healing.
3. prevent contamination from loose hair.
4. clear the wound of dried or excess blood.

161. Mixing different metals in the same ultrasonic cleaning cycle may result in:
1. spotting.
2. pitting.
3. corrosion.
4. staining.

162. Metzenbaum scissors have:
1. blunt tips with straight or curved blades.
2. short, thick jaws with serrated edges.
3. blunt tips with one blade terminating into a thin, curved hook.
4. pointed or blunt tips with straight or curved blades.

163. During a surgical procedure, which of the following can be used to ligate blood vessels or tissues?
1. Halsted mosquito forceps
2. Rochester-Pean forceps
3. Rochester-Carmalt forceps
4. Hemostatic forceps

164. When an animal is anesthetized prior to an oro-gastric intubation, a cuffed, tight-fitting endotra-cheal should be used because:
    1. this method will prevent aspiration of the administered material.
    2. animals will tolerate this tube better when under anesthesia.
    3. the chances of the tube being disrupted by movement are reduced.
    4. the use of this tube will allow for a shorter procedure time.

165. Schirmer's tear test is used to diagnose what ocular condition?
    1. Conjunctivitis
    2. Glaucoma
    3. Keratoconjunctivitis siccca
    4. Cherry eye

166. Neutrophils and monocytes travel to the site of a wound to remove foreign material, necrotic tissue, and bacteria in which phase of wound healing?
    1. Inflammatory
    2. Debridement
    3. Repair
    4. Maturation

167. When maintaining hemostasis for the surgeon, you should avoid:
    1. placing the suction tip near tissue.
    2. wiping the area with a gauze square.
    3. counting the gauze squares you used.
    4. cutting suture material after it is placed.

168. When washing surgical instruments, you should always use:
    1. chlorhexidine.
    2. a surgical scrub.
    3. a neutral pH cleanser.
    4. dish soap.

169. For which of the following patients should you exercise special care when applying isopropyl alcohol during a surgical scrub?
    1. German shepherd
    2. Boxer
    3. Chihuahua
    4. Bulldog

170. Nonfresh surgical milk may:
    1. lead to staining or corrosion.
    2. cause contamination of surgical instruments.
    3. decrease the lubrication of instruments.
    4. lead to spotting.

171. A tapered point suture needle would *most likely* be used on:
    1. skin.
    2. muscle.
    3. tendons.
    4. cartilage.

172. Which of the following is an example of self-retaining forceps?
    1. Russian tissue forceps
    2. Dressing forceps
    3. Allis tissue forceps
    4. Adson tissue forceps

173. You are giving instructions to a patient's owner about administering medication at home. The veterinarian's instructions say to give the patient eye drops "O.U. b.i.d." What do the veterinarian's instructions mean?
    1. Give the patient eye drops in both eyes once per day.
    2. Give the patient eye drops in the right eye once per day.
    3. Give the patient eye drops in both eyes twice per day.
    4. Give the patient eye drops in the right eye twice per day.

174. Which of the following patients should be admin-istered emetics to empty its stomach contents?
    1. A ferret that ingested a toxic plant and is unconscious
    2. A cat that ingested a corrosive toxin from its owner's garage
    3. A dog that ingested a full bottle of its owner's medication
    4. A rabbit that ingested some type of household chemical

175. Which of the following animals would most likely be classified in the "dead, dying, or euthanized" category during triage if it had a broken femur?
1. A dog
2. A cat
3. A horse
4. A rabbit

176. You are administering a shot in the scruff of a dog's neck. This type of injection is best described as:
1. intramuscular.
2. subcutaneous.
3. intravenous.
4. gastrointestinal.

177. You read a patient's chart that says the patient suffered a laceration from an accident. A laceration is best described as a wound that:
1. is characterized by the exposure of the dermis and is usually not serious.
2. does not show obvious signs on the skin's surface, but goes deep into the tissue.
3. includes major damage to the skin and other soft tissue and easily gets infected.
4. involves the rupture of a blood vessel below the skin's surface where blood pools.

178. A recumbent patient will be staying at your clinic. When caring for the recumbent patient, you should:
1. house the patient in a kennel big enough for it to move around in.
2. keep the patient far away from areas with lots of activity.
3. fill the patient's kennel with stiff or thin bedding.
4. clean and groom the patient on a daily basis.

179. Which of the following grooming instruments would work best for removing mats in an animal's coat?
1. Double-sided brush
2. Sticker brush
3. Metal comb
4. Hound glove

180. You are performing an examination of a canine patient and you measure his weight at 10 pounds. What is the dog's weight in kilograms?
1. 4.53 kilograms
2. 9.04 kilograms
3. 15.02 kilograms
4. 22.04 kilograms

181. Which of the following is a reason a patient would be immobilized by its bandages?
1. To prevent hemorrhaging at the site of a wound
2. To stop the patient from moving a fractured limb
3. To prevent against infection of the patient's injury
4. To stop or control swelling at the site of a wound

182. A simple fracture is a fracture in which the:
1. broken bone damages organs or vessels.
2. bone is broken into two pieces.
3. broken bone causes a wound on the skin.
4. bone is broken into more than two pieces.

183. Which of the following would contraindicate fluid therapy?
1. Constipation.
2. Pulmonary contusions.
3. Tachycardia.
4. Shock.

184. On an ECG, a progressive lengthening of the PR interval on successive beats accompanied by the occurrence of P waves without QRS complexes would indicate:
1. first-degree AV block.
2. Type I second-degree AV block.
3. Type II second-degree AV block.
4. third-degree AV block.

185. When administering a Schirmer's tear test, which of the following results would indicate a diagnosis of keratitis sicca in a feline patient?
1. 9 millimeters of moisture
2. 11 millimeters of moisture
3. 12 millimeters of moisture
4. 14 millimeters of moisture

186. What type of bandaging is used to stabilize a fracture prior to surgical repair?
1. Ehmer sling
2. Hobble
3. Velpeau sling
4. Robert Jones bandage

187. Which of the following drugs must be stored in a secure location, such as a locked cabinet or a safe?
1. Nystatin
2. Furosemide
3. Testosterone
4. Chlorpromazine

188. Chondrosarcoma is a malignant tumor of the:
1. bone
2. fibrous tissue
3. cartilage
4. blood vessels

189. Which of the following is a possible cause of sinus tachycardia?
1. Acidosis
2. Hypokalemia
3. Hyperthyroidism
4. Ventricular concentric hypertrophy

190. A fluid-filled blister measuring 0.3 centimeter is called a:
1. bulla.
2. wheal.
3. papule.
4. vesicle.

191. When used for wound lavage, povidone-iodine solution:
1. has an immediate microbial effect and a long-term residual effect.
2. can damage tissues because of its foaming effect.
3. is inactivated by exudates, blood, and organic material.
4. should be used for irrigation only once.

192. When performing venipuncture through the jugular vein, the patient should be placed in:
1. right lateral recumbency.
2. dorsal recumbency.
3. left lateral recumbency.
4. sternal recumbency.

193. You can ensure an adequate blood flow during venipuncture by:
1. applying alcohol to the puncture site.
2. occluding the vein.
3. inserting the needle with the bevel facing downward.
4. pulling back the plunger as quickly as possible.

194. You are instructing a patient's owner about collecting a urine sample. You should instruct the owner to:
1. take the sample right before the animal goes to sleep.
2. collect all the urine the patient expresses during one bathroom break.
3. bring in the sample as soon as possible after it's taken.
4. give the animal as much water as possible before taking the sample.

195. A veterinary technician is treating a dog with a mandible that is wider than the maxilla in the area near the premolars. This condition is referred to as a:
1. rostral crossbite.
2. caudal crossbite.
3. distoclusion.
4. mesioclusion.

196. A patient in your clinic had a 10% change in its white blood cell count from one day to the next. These findings are most likely:
1. significant because a 10% change is large enough to cause concern.
2. insignificant because a 10% change is too low to cause concern.
3. significant because even slight changes in white blood cell counts are serious.
4. insignificant because any changes in white blood cell counts are unimportant.

197. For which of the following diseases would a veterinary technician most likely conduct a capillary refill time (CRT) test?
1. Cancer
2. Liver disease
3. Cataracts
4. Heart disease

198. Which level is generally tested and analyzed with potassium during a chemical panel?
1. Cholesterol
2. Sodium
3. Calcium
4. SGPT

199. Which of the following materials would be thrown in the regular waste, rather than the biomedical waste?
1. A needle covered in blood from a healthy rabbit
2. Rubber tubing covered in saliva from a raccoon with tuberculosis
3. A scalpel covered with blood from a healthy bird
4. Paper covered in urine from a cat infected with ear mites

200. Which teeth are used primarily for cutting and nibbling?
1. Incisors
2. Canines
3. Premolars
4. Molars

ANSWER KEY AND EXPLANATIONS

1. 3	41. 2	81. 2	121. 4	161. 3
2. 2	42. 3	82. 2	122. 2	162. 4
3. 3	43. 3	83. 4	123. 3	163. 4
4. 2	44. 1	84. 2	124. 2	164. 1
5. 2	45. 2	85. 2	125. 4	165. 3
6. 3	46. 3	86. 3	126. 4	166. 2
7. 4	47. 2	87. 3	127. 2	167. 2
8. 4	48. 3	88. 3	128. 2	168. 3
9. 3	49. 2	89. 1	129. 3	169. 3
10. 4	50. 2	90. 2	130. 3	170. 2
11. 4	51. 2	91. 4	131. 2	171. 2
12. 2	52. 4	92. 3	132. 1	172. 3
13. 4	53. 2	93. 1	133. 1	173. 3
14. 3	54. 2	94. 3	134. 1	174. 3
15. 3	55. 2	95. 4	135. 1	175. 3
16. 2	56. 1	96. 2	136. 4	176. 2
17. 2	57. 1	97. 3	137. 4	177. 3
18. 2	58. 3	98. 2	138. 2	178. 4
19. 3	59. 2	99. 2	139. 1	179. 3
20. 3	60. 4	100. 1	140. 4	180. 1
21. 2	61. 2	101. 4	141. 1	181. 2
22. 4	62. 4	102. 4	142. 2	182. 2
23. 1	63. 2	103. 3	143. 2	183. 2
24. 3	64. 3	104. 1	144. 3	184. 2
25. 3	65. 2	105. 3	145. 4	185. 1
26. 4	66. 4	106. 3	146. 2	186. 4
27. 1	67. 1	107. 4	147. 1	187. 3
28. 4	68. 3	108. 3	148. 4	188. 3
29. 3	69. 2	109. 1	149. 3	189. 3
30. 3	70. 4	110. 2	150. 2	190. 4
31. 1	71. 4	111. 3	151. 2	191. 3
32. 3	72. 1	112. 1	152. 4	192. 4
33. 2	73. 1	113. 4	153. 3	193. 2
34. 4	74. 3	114. 2	154. 4	194. 3
35. 2	75. 3	115. 3	155. 4	195. 2
36. 3	76. 3	116. 4	156. 2	196. 2
37. 3	77. 4	117. 4	157. 1	197. 4
38. 4	78. 1	118. 2	158. 3	198. 2
39. 1	79. 2	119. 4	159. 3	199. 4
40. 2	80. 2	120. 1	160. 3	200. 1

1. **The correct answer is 3.** Nitrous oxide should not be used with a rebreathing system because of the risk of oxygen depletion and nitrous oxide buildup. Choices 1, 2, and 4—halothane, isoflurane, and desflurane—can all be safely used with a rebreathing system.

2. **The correct answer is 2.** It is recommended that you bury the needle in the veins of medium and large breeds of dog—such as the golden retriever—when taking a blood sample. This will prevent the needle from slipping out of the vein if the patient moves during the procedure. Persian cats, Oriental cats, and Pomeranians (choices 1, 3, and 4) are incorrect because these animals are smaller, and only about half the needle should be buried while taking blood samples from them.

3. **The correct answer is 3.** A gastrointestinal obstruction would contraindicate the administration of morphine as a preanesthetic because morphine often results in an increased risk of vomiting. Preexisting tachycardia (choice 1), liver disease (choice 2), and respiratory disease (choice 4) would not interfere with the administration of morphine, so those choices are incorrect.

4. **The correct answer is 2.** Reports of contagious or zoonotic diseases may not always be subject to the confidentiality requirements of a patient's medical record because of the risk to others around the patient. Choices 1, 3, and 4 are all subject to confidentiality requirements. Such information can only be released with proper consent.

5. **The correct answer is 2.** An abscess is best described as a collection of material from a bacterial infection in the tooth. An oronasal fistula is an abnormal communication between the oral and nasal cavities (choice 1). An impaction is a tooth that is unable to break through the gum surface, so choice 3 is incorrect. Choice 4 is incorrect because a cavity is a hole in the tooth.

6. **The correct answer is 3.** Bisacodyl is a laxative and would be administered to a patient experiencing constipation. Oxazepam, choice 1, is a type of appetite stimulant often used in cats. Ranitidine, choice 2, is an anti-ulcer medication. Apomorphine, choice 4, is an emetic that would be used to induce vomiting. Therefore, choices 1, 2, and 4 are incorrect.

7. **The correct answer is 4.** Cholinergic drugs stimulate the parasympathetic nervous system. Choice 1 is incorrect because opioids and other drugs decrease the sensation of pain. Beta-blockers are drugs that block the action of adrenaline at beta-adrenergic receptors, so choice 2 is not correct. Choice 3 is incorrect because mydriatic drugs dilate the pupil.

8. **The correct answer is 4.** When discarding a used needle, you should handle the needle carefully and dispose of it in the appropriate container. Used needles could harbor dangerous bacteria and diseases, so handling the needle as little as possible is advised. Destroying the needle, choice 1, is not correct because when you break the needle, its contents could go into the air you're breathing. Separating the needle and the syringe, choice 2, is incorrect because this would cause you to handle the needle longer than necessary, increasing the risk of your harming yourself. Recapping the needle, choice 3, is incorrect because you could potentially stick yourself with the needle.

9. **The correct answer is 3.** Based on the given signs and symptoms, the patient is currently 10–12% dehydrated. An animal with a lower degree of dehydration, choices 1 and 2, would present with fewer and less severe symptoms. An animal with a higher degree of dehydration, choice 4, would present with more severe symptoms and could be fatal.

10. **The correct answer is 4.** Gastric dilation and volvulus is a life-threatening condition. Dogs experiencing this condition repeatedly look at or even bite their abdomen, which is typically distended. These dogs also retch without vomiting. This bloating can result in decreased blood flow and the loss of stomach tissue if it is not treated immediately. Many times, the animal needs surgery to relieve the pressure. Choices 1, 2, and 3 are incorrect because the condition is a true emergency. An example of a minor emergency would be a burn, while an example of a serious emergency would be a fracture.

11. **The correct answer is 4.** Barium is considered an insoluble positive contrast media. Barium can absorb more X-rays than bone, so it will appear whiter on radiographs. Choices 1 and 3 are incorrect

because barium is insoluble, not soluble. Choice 2 is incorrect because barium is a positive, not negative, contrast media.

12. **The correct answer is 2.** Trichiasis, which refers to ingrown hairs that affect the eye, is most common among poodles. English bulldogs, pugs, and cocker spaniels are not commonly affected by trichiasis, so choices 1, 3, and 4 are incorrect.

13. **The correct answer is 4.** Jacobs chucks are surgical instruments used to advance pin placement. Rongeurs are used to break up and remove bone, so choice 1 is incorrect. Choice 2 is not correct because verbrugge forceps and reduction forceps are used to hold bone fragments in reduction. Bone-cutting forceps or osteotomes are used to cut through bone, making choice 3 incorrect.

14. **The correct answer is 3.** Purchasing the most affordable medications possible would be considered a poor inventory control practice because, although careful spending is important, simply buying the cheapest products available may endanger the welfare of your patients. Choices 1, 2, and 4 are all acceptable inventory control practices.

15. **The correct answer is 3.** Mannitol, a diuretic, would be used to reduce intracranial pressure. Choice 1, atropine, is used for cardiac support. Choice 2, pimobendan, is used to manage congestive heart failure. Choice 4, prazosin, is used to treat functional urethral obstructions. Therefore, choices 1, 2, and 4 are incorrect.

16. **The correct answer is 2.** Guaifenesin crosses the placental barrier, but has little effect on the fetus. Choice 1 is not correct because guaifenesin has some effect on the fetus. Choices 3 and 4 are incorrect because guaifenesin does cross the placental barrier.

17. **The correct answer is 2.** A healthy horse should have a white blood cell count ranging from 6–12. Choice 1 is incorrect because it indicates the white blood cell count of a cow. Choice 3 is incorrect because it indicates the white blood cell count of a dog. Choice 4 is incorrect because it indicates the white blood cell count of a thoroughbred.

18. **The correct answer is 2.** Veterinary dentists use a shepherd's hook to detect external odontoclastic resorptive lesions in a cat. Periodontal probes are use to measure depth in the mouth, so choice 1 is incorrect. A curette is used to scrape the teeth, so choice 3 is incorrect. Choice 4 is not correct because a sickle scaler is used to remove deposits from the teeth.

19. **The correct answer is 3.** Patient movement during the X-ray process may result in diminished radiographic detail. Ineffective filtration, low subject contrast, and negative contrast use will not result in diminished radiographic detail, so choices 1, 2, and 4 are incorrect.

20. **The correct answer is 3.** When extracting a blood sample from the lateral saphenous vein, canine patients should be placed in lateral recumbency. When extracting from the jugular or cephalic veins, choices 1 and 2, the patient should be placed in sternal recumbency. Blood sample extraction from the femoral vein, choice 4, is generally performed only on feline patients.

21. **The correct answer is 2.** The correct method of restraining a patient for a blood sample collection from the cephalic vein would be to place the fingers of one hand behind the patient's elbow to extend the front leg. The method described in choice 1 would be used for an extraction from the jugular vein. The method described in choice 3 would be used for an extraction from the lateral saphenous vein. The method described in choice 4 would be used for an extraction from the femoral vein of a feline patient. Therefore, choices 1, 3, and 4 are incorrect.

22. **The correct answer is 4.** Digoxin, a positive inotrope, is designed to provide long-term maintenance of contractibility. Choice 1, dobutamine, is used for short-term maintenance of contractibility. Choice 2, hydralazine, is used to dilate blood vessels. Choice 3, propranolol, is used to block Beta-receptors.

23. **The correct answer is 1.** This would be an accurate description of a Brown-Adson forceps. This type of forceps, which also features wide blade sides, is used with delicate tissue. This description would not be accurate for any of the other choices.

24. **The correct answer is 3.** Feline blood donors must weigh at least 10 pounds. A feline blood

donor under 10 pounds might not have an adequate blood volume to withstand donation, so choices 1 and 2 are incorrect. Choice 4 is incorrect because a feline can weigh less than 12 pounds, just not less than 10 pounds.

25. **The correct answer is 3.** Sarcoptic mange is a parasitic condition caused by Sarcoptes mites, which results in the symptoms the patient is experiencing. Choice 1, demodectic mange, presents with non-itchy patches of red scaly ringworm-like lesions around the face and front legs. Walking dandruff, choice 2, results in small, white insects on the animal's hair. Fleas, choice 4, presents with crusty skin, itching, flea dirt, and alopecia.

26. **The correct answer is 4.** You should never wait to address a conflict, as this may be likely to cause the problem to worsen. Taking any action to achieve conflict resolution, such as having a face-to-face conversation (choice 1), bringing the matter up at a staff meeting (choice 2), or filing a written complaint (choice 3) would be more effective than taking no immediate action at all.

27. **The correct answer is 1.** Azaperone is a type of butyrophenone that is commonly used as a preanesthetic for aggressive pigs. This use is unique to swine, so choices 2, 3, and 4 are incorrect.

28. **The correct answer is 4.** The rinse bath serves to stop the process of development and prevent contamination of the fixer. Choices 1 and 2 are incorrect because the developer begins the developing process and converts the exposed silver halide crystals to metallic silver. The fixer clears away the underexposed silver halide crystals, so choice 3 is incorrect.

29. **The correct answer is 3.** Propofol would be the most appropriate agent to use for anesthetizing a greyhound. This particular anesthetic agent is the primary means of anesthetizing lean-bodied animals. None of the other choices are specifically used in this circumstance.

30. **The correct answer is 3.** When you are preparing a large dog for surgery, at least 4 inches of hair on either side of the midline must be removed. Choices 1 and 2 may indicate that too little hair

should be removed, and choice 4 indicates that too much hair should be removed.

31. **The correct answer is 1.** The buccal surface is the surface area of a tooth that faces towards the cheek. Choice 2 refers to the surface facing towards the lips. Choice 3 refers to the surface facing the nose. Choice 4 refers to the chewing surface.

32. **The correct answer is 3.** Surgical instruments that have been properly protected with wrapping material and stored on an open shelf can remain sterile for up to three weeks. This is the only accurate choice.

33. **The correct answer is 2.** The normal sulcus depth for a cat is less than 1 millimeter. Sulcus depth measuring between 1 and 3 millimeters is normal in dogs. Choice 1 is incorrect because that depth is too low. Choices 3 and 4 are incorrect because those depths are too high.

34. **The correct answer is 4.** Chemosis, which is edema of the ocular conjunctiva, is a common sign of overhydration. Lowered blood pressure, decreased lung sounds, and fatigue are not symptoms of overhydration, so choices 1, 2, and 3 are incorrect.

35. **The correct answer is 2.** Using hydrogen peroxide for wound lavage can lead to tissue damage as a result of its foaming effect. None of the other substances would risk tissue damage.

36. **The correct answer is 3.** A professional organization specializing in veterinary medicine is the best place to find answers about professional ethics questions for veterinary technicians. Many of these organizations even have codes of ethics, which they maintain all veterinary medical professionals should follow. Choice 1 is incorrect because questions of professional ethics often require input from others. Choice 2 is incorrect because ethical standards almost always exceed the standards set by laws. Choice 4 is incorrect because a friend who doesn't work in veterinary medicine most likely doesn't fully understand the technician's ethical problem.

37. **The correct answer is 3.** EDTA is the most commonly used anticoagulant for blood testing. Of the various anticoagulants used in blood testing, EDTA is the most effective and least likely to interfere with the results. Oxalate, choice 1, is no

longer used for blood testing. Heparin, choice 2, is a natural coagulant in the body and, as a result may interfere with some blood tests. Sodium citrate, choice 4, may interfere with chemical tests or shrink cells.

38. **The correct answer is 4.** Auranofin is an immunosuppressant agent used in veterinary medicine. Choice 1 is incorrect because dextran is used as a fluid replacement. Choice 2, lactulose, is incorrect because it is a laxative. Choice 3 is not correct because interferon is an immunostimulant.

39. **The correct answer is 1.** The denser a body part is, the whiter it will appear on an X-ray. Choices 2, 3, and 4 are all incorrect because the denser body parts don't appear darker, grayer, or foggier than less dense parts.

40. **The correct answer is 2.** Hip dysplasia is a genetic disease of the hip joint in dogs. Since large dog breeds are more prone to this disease, a mastiff would be at a higher risk for developing hip dysplasia than smaller dog breeds such as a Chihuahua, Jack Russell terrier, and greyhound.

41. **The correct answer is 2.** X-rays should always be taken from at least two angles to ensure the most accurate diagnosis. An X-ray taken from only one angle may not offer a fully accurate view of the problem. Although X-rays could be taken from more than two angles, this is generally not necessary.

42. **The correct answer is 3.** A lethal dose of methohexital is only two to three times its normal anesthetic dosage. Generally thiopental, pentobarbital, and phenobarbital are not lethal at dosages two to three times their normal anesthetic dose. Therefore, choices 1, 2, and 4 are incorrect.

43. **The correct answer is 3.** The fresh gas flow rate for a non-rebreathing system should be set between 130 to 300 mL/kg/min. Choices 1 and 2 are incorrect because these flow rates would be too low and could result in rebreathing of exhaled gases. Choice 4 would be incorrect because that flow rate is too high.

44. **The correct answer is 1.** Polydioxanone is a synthetic absorbable suture material. Choices 2, 3, and 4 are all nonabsorbable suture materials.

45. **The correct answer is 2.** The patient's dental condition would be referred to as an anterior crossbite. Choice 1 refers to a malocclusion in which the mandible is wider than the maxilla in the premolar area. Choice 3 refers to a malocclusion in which the mandibular teeth are distal to their maxillary equivalents. Choice 4 refers to a malocclusion where the mandibular teeth occlude rostral to their maxillary counterparts.

46. **The correct answer is 3.** Rabbits develop only one set of teeth during their lifetimes. Choices 1, 2, and 4 all develop both deciduous (primary) and permanent teeth.

47. **The correct answer is 2.** Medications delivered intraosseously are injected into the bone cavity. Choice 1 (the skin) describes a subcutaneous injection. Choice 3 (a muscle) describes an intramuscular injection. Choice 4 (a blood vessel) describes an intravenous injection.

48. **The correct answer is 3.** A gaping wound is a condition a technician would most likely categorize as a serious emergency. Bee stings, minor burns, and even abscesses would all be minor emergencies that wouldn't require immediate assistance. Choices 1, 2, and 4 are incorrect as the owner can treat many of these conditions at home.

49. **The correct answer is 2.** If diazepam is accidently administered perivascularly, a veterinary technician should slowly inject sterile saline into the injection site to dilute the drug. Choice 1 is incorrect because technicians should never rapidly inject saline. Choices 3 and 4 are incorrect because the site should be numbed with an external cream, not an injected drug.

50. **The correct answer is 2.** Catgut, also known as surgical gut, is made from the submucosal layer of sheep intestines. Choices 1, 3, and 4 are incorrect because this suture material is not made from the intestines of cats, dogs, or cattle.

51. **The correct answer is 2.** Ketoconazole is a type of antimicrobial drug that inhibits nucleic acid production, thus interfering with DNA/RNA synthesis. Choices 1 and 4, penicillin and amoxicillin, are antimicrobial that disrupts the development of microbial cell walls. Tetracycline (choice 3) is an antimicrobial that interferes with microbial protein synthesis.

52. The correct answer is 4. Etodolac is an NSAID. Betamethasone, choice 1, is a corticosteroid. Choice 2, hyaluronate, is a glycosaminoglycan. Methocarbamol, choice 3, is a muscle relaxant.

53. The correct answer is 2. Exhausted fixer solution can lead to a yellow radiograph. Choice 1 can lead to black marks on the radiograph. Choice 3 can lead to white marks or clear areas on the radiograph. Choice 4 can lead to a brittle finished radiograph.

54. The correct answer is 2. A lavender Vacutainer top indicates EDTA without other additives. A red Vacutainer top, choice 1, indicates a Vacutainer with no additives at all. A light blue Vacutainer top, choice 3, indicates sodium citrate. A dark blue Vacutainer top, choice 4, indicates both EDTA and heparin.

55. The correct answer is 2. Cyclohexamines cause an increase in ocular pressure, which could be dangerous for patients with glaucoma or perforation of the eye chamber. Glaucoma would not contraindicate the use of etomidate, fentanyl, or propofol.

56. The correct answer is 1. Sevoflurane is ideal for use with avian species because it has a rapid, smooth induction and recovery, which minimizes patient stress. Choices 2, 3, and 4 are incorrect because these inhaled anesthetics are not so effective for avian species.

57. The correct answer is 1. A lower grid ratio would indicate that less scatter radiation is absorbed. The higher the grid ratio, the more scatter and primary radiation is absorbed. Therefore, choice 2 is incorrect. Choices 3 and 4 are incorrect because the grid ratio does not affect how much radiation is being emitted.

58. The correct answer is 3. Pentastarch is classified as a colloid. Hartmann's solution, Lactated Ringer's solution, and saline are crystalloids, so choices 1, 2, and 4 are incorrect.

59. The correct answer is 2. Babesia canis is a canine blood parasite. Choices 1, 3, and 4 are incorrect because Ehrlichia canis, Ehrlichia platy, and Borrelia burgdorferi are all rickettsial diseases.

60. The correct answer is 4. Finochietto retractors are commonly used during thoracic surgery to retract the ribs. Abdominal surgeries, choice 1, may involve the use of Balfour retractors. Neurosurgery and orthopedic surgeries, choices 2 and 3, may both involve the use of Gelpi retractors or Weitlander retractors.

61. The correct answer is 2. Quantum mottle is a loss of radiographic detail common with faster screens because of unevenly distributed phosphor crystals within the intensifying screen. Choice 1, penumbra, is a loss of detail because of geometric unsharpness. Choice 3, structure mottle, is the loss of detail due to phosphor variations in the intensifying screen. Choice 4, radiographic mottle, is the loss of detail due to the size of the individual silver halide crystals.

62. The correct answer is 4. Small volume blood samples are usually extracted from the tail vein in cows. The milk vein, choice 1, is a secondary option for bovine small blood samples, but this location presents an increased risk of hematoma. The jugular vein, choice 2, would be used to obtain a large volume sample. The caudal auricular vein, choice 3, is the common site of small volume blood sampling in pigs.

63. The correct answer is 2. Myelography is a diagnostic imaging test in which a dye is injected into the spinal column in order to highlight small changes in the spinal cord. Choice 1, nuclear scintigraphy, involves the injection of a radioactive compound that travels through the bloodstream and targets specific organs. Choice 3, an MRI, is a diagnostic imaging test that utilizes magnetic fields and radio waves to produce detailed body images. Choice 4, endoscopy, is a diagnostic imaging test most often used to diagnose digestive issues.

64. The correct answer is 3. Boxers are most commonly associated with gingival hyperplasia, which is a gingival thickening precipitated by chronic inflammation. None of the breeds in choices 1, 2, or 4 are commonly associated with this condition.

65. The correct answer is 2. Melanoma is the most common type of oral tumor among dogs. Fibrosarcoma, choice 1, is the third most common canine oral tumor. Osteosarcoma, choice 3, is the least common oral tumor among dogs. Squamous cell carcinoma, choice 4, is the second most common canine oral tumor.

66. **The correct answer is 4.** Cats with type AB blood may receive any type of feline blood. Cats with type A or B blood, however, may only receive their own blood type.

67. **The correct answer is 1.** Halothane, an inhaled anesthetic, may result in an increase in cerebrospinal fluid pressure. Choices 2, 3, and 4 are incorrect because guaifenesin, isoflurane, and sevoflurane are not known for increasing cerebrospinal fluid pressure.

68. **The correct answer is 3.** A 22 gauge is the most commonly used needle size for venipuncture in cats and small dogs. Choices 1 and 2, 18 and 20 gauge needles, are incorrect because these sizes are normally used for larger animals. A 24 gauge needle, choice 4, may be used less commonly for cats and small dogs.

69. **The correct answer is 2.** Xylamine is an emetic drug used to induce vomiting in cats. Choice 1, chlorpromazine, is an antiemetic that would prevent vomiting. Choice 3, metoclopramide, works to increase gastric motility. Choice 4, aminopentamide, is an antispasmodic that is used to treat spasms or cramps in the stomach, intestines, or bladder.

70. **The correct answer is 4.** The surface on which you could safely use bleach is the linoleum floors because the bleach would disinfect surface without harming it. Choice 1 is incorrect because bleach is a tissue irritant, and should not be used on animals or humans. Choices 2 and 3 are incorrect because bleach can be corrosive to metal.

71. **The correct answer is 4.** Ondansetron is used to treat refractory vomiting, which is a frequent side effect of chemotherapy. Choices 1 and 2, dimenhydrinate and meclizine, are primarily used to treat motion sickness. Choice 3, metoclopramide, is a promotility agent used to inhibit gastroesophageal reflux.

72. **The correct answer is 1.** Nylon rope toys can cause gingival trauma if the gingiva is sliced by fine nylon threads. Dried hooves and nylon chew bones, choices 2 and 3, can lead to slab fractures. Rawhide strips, choice 4, are generally considered safe and may actually serve to remove debris from between teeth.

73. **The correct answer is 1.** Radiographic detail can be increased by increasing the source-image distance. This will decrease magnification and the level of penumbra. Decreasing the source-image distance, choice 2, would have the opposite effect. Increasing the object-film distance, choice 3, would increase magnification and the level of penumbra, also the opposite effect. Increasing the kVp level, choice 4, may lead to overpenetration, which would cause an overly dark film with grayed bones.

74. **The correct answer is 3.** Histopathology, which is the biopsy of part or all of a mass for analysis, is the definitive means of diagnosing a malignant tumor. Cytology, choice 1, is used to determine the cell morphology of a tumor and can also be diagnostic. Radiography and serum chemistry profile, choices 2 and 4, are often used as part of the patient's evaluation, but are not necessarily diagnostic.

75. **The correct answer is 3.** Improperly applied bandages can cause many problems for animals, including tissue necrosis. The other choices are incorrect because wound drainage (choice 1), immobilization of a limb (choice 2), and wound debridement (choice 4) are all positive effects of properly applied bandages.

76. **The correct answer is 3.** The minimum weight for a canine blood donor is 55 pounds. Choices 1 and 2 (25 and 45 pounds) are under the minimum weight requirement. Dogs this small may not have the adequate blood volume to withstand blood donation. Choice 4, 65 pounds, exceeds the minimum weight for donation.

77. **The correct answer is 4.** Guinea pigs must be sedated or anesthetized for venipuncture. The species in choices 1, 2, and 3—Mongolian gerbil, mouse, and rat—can all tolerate venipuncture without sedation or anesthesia.

78. **The correct answer is 1.** Clindamycin should not be administered to rabbits because of potential gastrointestinal side effects. This medication should also be avoided with hamsters, guinea pigs, chinchillas, horses, and ruminants for the same

reason. None of the antimicrobials in choices 2, 3, or 4 have this side effect.

79. **The correct answer is 2.** Dantrolene should be used in the event of malignant hyperthermia. Calcium EDTA, choice 1, should be used in the event of lead poisoning. Pamidronate, choice 3, should be used in the event of cholecalciferol toxicosis. Atropine, choice 4, should be used in the event of organophosphate toxicity. Therefore, choices 1, 3, and 4 are incorrect.

80. **The correct answer is 2.** In smooth inductions, the patient will normally skip Stage 2 and transition directly from Stage 1 to Stage 3. Stages 1 and 3, choices 1 and 3, always occur. Stage 4, choice 4, does not normally occur and, as it is the final stage, it cannot be bypassed.

81. **The correct answer is 2.** A Number 11 blade would be used with a Number 3 handle for severing ligaments during a small animal surgical procedure. A Number 10 blade, choice 1, is used to incise skin. A Number 12 blade, choice 3, is used to lance abscesses. A Number 15 blade, choice 4, would be used to make precise, small, or curved incisions. Therefore, choices 1, 3, and 4 are incorrect.

82. **The correct answer is 2.** A high dose of xylazine could be dangerous for a ruminant. Ruminant species receiving high doses of xylazine may experience decreased oxygen exchange. None of the preanesthetics in choices 1, 3, or 4 would cause this potential side effect.

83. **The correct answer is 4.** An excessively high level of vitamin D is thought to be a possible contributing factor in the development of feline odontoclastic resorptive lesions. Canned cat foods frequently contain excess vitamin D, which can lead to hypervitaminosis D. It is believed that this condition may be associated with the development of feline odontoclastic resorptive lesions. None of the vitamins in choices 1, 2, or 3 is linked to feline odontoclastic resorptive lesions.

84. **The correct answer is 2.** A tourniquet immobilizes a limb and cuts off blood flow to that limb; if the tourniquet is left on too long, the limb could die from a lack of blood flow. The longest a tourniquet should be used is 20 minutes. Choice 1 is not correct because tourniquets can be used safely for more than 5 minutes. Choices 3 and 4 are incorrect because 40 and 60 minutes are too long to keep on a tourniquet.

85. **The correct answer is 2.** Lagomorphs, or rabbits, do not have canines. They do, however, have incisors, premolars, and molars, so choices 1, 3, and 4 are incorrect.

86. **The correct answer is 3.** Tooth overgrowth is commonly associated with vitamin C deficiency in guinea pigs. None of the conditions in choices 1, 2, or 4 are connected to vitamin C.

87. **The correct answer is 3.** Slow speed screens are designed to produce optimum detail with little regard to exposure time. Medium speed screens produce average quality resolution radiographs with relatively low exposures, so choice 1 is incorrect. Fast speed screens are used when increased patient penetration is needed and normally have a thicker phosphor layer, so choices 2 and 4 are incorrect.

88. **The correct answer is 3.** Increased cerebrospinal fluid pressure is a cause of sinus bradycardia. Hyperthyroidism, anemia, and reduced cardiac output are all potential causes of sinus tachycardia, not sinus bradycardia, so choices 1, 2, and 4 are incorrect.

89. **The correct answer is 1.** Manual compression of the bladder would be an appropriate method for examining solute concentration in urine. Although manual compression of the bladder would not provide a sterile urine sample for urinalysis or culture, urine collected in this manner could be examined for solute concentration and other purposes. Cystocentesis would be an appropriate method for relieving bladder distention due to obstruction, so choice 2 is incorrect. Catheterization or cystocentesis would be appropriate methods for collecting a sterile urine sample for urinalysis and culture, so choice 3 is incorrect. Catheterization is an appropriate method for clearing a urethral obstruction, so choice 4 is incorrect.

90. **The correct answer is 2.** Halsted mosquito forceps have transverse serrations covering the entire jaw length. Kelly forceps have distal transverse grooves (choice 1). Crile forceps have complete transverse grooves (choice 3). Rochester-Carmalt forceps

have longitudinal grooves and distal transverse grooves (choice 4). Choices 1, 3, and 4 are incorrect.

91. **The correct answer is 4.** When cutting and dissecting dense tissue, a surgeon would most likely use Mayo scissors. Choice 1, Metzenbaum scissors, are used to cut and dissect delicate tissue. Choice 2, Iris scissors, are most often used for intraocular surgery. Choice 3, Spencer scissors, are suture removal scissors. Therefore, choices 1, 2, and 3 are incorrect.

92. **The correct answer is 3.** Miconazole is used to treat fungal ophthalmic infections. Choices 1, 2, and 4 are incorrect because miconazole is not used to treat these problems. Nystatin is used to treat gastrointestinal and skin Candida infections (choice 1). Terbinafine is used to treat dermatophytosis or avian mycoses (choice 2). Sulfasalazine is used to treat inflammatory bowel disease (choice 4).

93. **The correct answer is 1.** Halothane has the highest rate of metabolization, with about 40% of the inhaled gas being metabolized, rather than exhaled. Sevoflurane (choice 2) is about 3% metabolized. Nitrous oxide (choice 3) is about 0.0004% metabolized. Desflurane (choice 4) is about 0.02% metabolized.

94. **The correct answer is 3.** Blood samples that need to be allowed to clot should be placed in a Vacutainer with a red top. The red top indicates that there are no anticoagulants or other additives already in the vial. Choices 1, 2, and 4 all indicate that the vial contains some form of anticoagulant or other additive, so these choices are not correct.

95. **The correct answer is 4.** Etomidate is particularly useful for patients with cardiac disease because it does not affect cardiac output, respiratory rate, or blood pressure. Cyclohexamines, choice 1, produce cardiovascular stimulation. Barbiturates, choice 2, can depress respiration and cardiovascular activity. Propofol, choice 3, can have various cardiovascular side effects.

96. **The correct answer is 2.** The reduction of orally administered drugs in the liver is known as the first-pass effect. When an orally administered drug is taken, it immediately travels to the liver and may be reduced or removed before reaching the bloodstream. Perfusion is the passage of blood through tissue vessels, so choice 1 is incorrect. Diffusion, choice 3, is incorrect because it is the process of spreading to and from various areas of concentration. Choice 4, second-pass metabolism, is incorrect because the term doesn't exist.

97. **The correct answer is 3.** When the needle is removed from the vein, you should immediately apply pressure over the venipuncture site. This will provide hemostasis and stop the bleeding. Choice 1, placing the sample into a Vacutainer, should happen after you apply pressure to the site. Choice 2, stopping compression of the vein, should occur before the needle is removed. Choice 4, releasing the patient from restrain, should not occur before hemostasis has been achieved.

98. **The correct answer is 2.** A patient with fever, anemia, heart murmur, and moderate dehydration would be considered a Category III patient. This patient would be deemed to be at moderate risk. A Category II patient, choice 1, would be deemed to be at slight risk. A Category IV patient, choice 3, would be deemed to be at high risk. A Category V patient, choice 4, would be deemed to be at extreme risk.

99. **The correct answer is 2.** Uveitis is an inflammation of the eye's middle vascular layer. Keratoconjunctivitis is decreased tear production and corneal film, so choice 1 is incorrect. Keratitis is corneal inflammation, so choice 2 is incorrect. Strabismus is the squinting or crossing of the eyes, so choice 4 is incorrect.

100. **The correct answer is 1.** When performing a surgical scrub, begin at the incision and work outward in a circular motion. This is the most effective means of cleaning and sanitizing the area of the incision. Choices 2, 3, and 4 are all incorrect as they are not so effective in preventing infection.

101. **The correct answer is 4.** In this scenario, the most appropriate treatment would be to administer milk and monitor. Drain cleaner is a caustic substance, so any induced vomiting could lead to further esophageal damage, so choice 1 is incorrect. Choice 2 is incorrect because activated charcoal may make it difficult to properly examine the GI tract. Choice 3 is an antidiarrheal and would not be an appropriate treatment.

102. **The correct answer is 4.** Canine blood donors must wait at least twelve days after a vaccination before they may donate again. This waiting period is due to the effects of vaccination on platelets and endothelial functions. Choices 2 and 3 are incorrect because they do not allow enough time for a dog's system to return to normal function. Choice 1 is incorrect because it is a longer period than is necessary.

103. **The correct answer is 3.** Newborn animals must be kept in facilities with temperatures of 75°–80°F for the first ten days of their lives. On the eleventh day, technicians can decrease the temperature of the room by a few degrees. During the fourth week, the newborns are then exposed to average room temperatures. Choices 1 and 2 are incorrect because the temperature ranges in these options are too cool for newborn animals. Choice 4 is incorrect because this temperature range is too warm.

104. **The correct answer is 1.** Distichiasis results in a second row of eyelashes. Trichiasis is ingrown eyelashes, so choice 2 is incorrect. Choice 3 is incorrect because hypertrophy is glandular tissue that projects beyond the haw. Choice 4 is incorrect because strabismus is the squinting or the crossing of the eyes.

105. **The correct answer is 3.** Doyen intestinal forceps are self-retaining forceps commonly used for holding bowels. Allis tissue forceps, choice 1, are self-retaining and have intermeshing teeth that may cause damage to delicate tissues. Choice 2, Babcock intestinal forceps, are like Allis tissue forceps, but have no gripping teeth. Choice 4, Ferguson angiotribe forceps, are also self-retaining and help to hold large bundles of tissue.

106. **The correct answer is 3.** Inserting the needle upwards toward the patient is an appropriate means of ensuring a successful venipuncture. This method helps to facilitate the flow of incoming blood and prevents occlusions by the vein. Choice 1, inserting the needle downward toward the patient, would have the opposite affect and may make collecting a sample more difficult. Choice 2, retracting the syringe plunger as quickly as possible, could cause the vein to collapse due to significant negative pressure. Choice 4, fully retracting the syringe plunger immediately upon puncture, is incorrect because you should retract the plunger only slightly at first, to ensure that the needle is actually in the vein.

107. **The correct answer is 4.** Etomidate is dangerous to use on horses and cattle because it can lead to severe muscle rigidity or seizures in these species. Fentanyl, propofol, and guaifenesin are incorrect because these drugs do not cause complications for horses and cattle.

108. **The correct answer is 3.** When packing a biopsy sample for shipping, you should add an appropriate fluid to the container to soak the sample. Biopsy samples must remain moist while they are shipped. Choice 1 is incorrect because biopsy samples should remain moist, not dry, during shipping. Choice 2 is incorrect because freezing biopsy samples can sometimes alter test results. Choice 4 is not correct because biopsy samples shouldn't be heated before they are shipped.

109. **The correct answer is 1.** Sevoflurane can result in a lessened or absent version of the hangover effect that normally accompanies inhaled anesthetics. Choices 2, 3, and 4 can cause a hangover effect when used.

110. **The correct answer is 2.** A drug with a high therapeutic index has a low toxicity level. Choice 1 is incorrect because drugs with high therapeutic indexes have low, not high, toxicity levels. Choices 3 and 4 are incorrect because therapeutic indexes aren't created based on side effects or potential benefits of drugs.

111. **The correct answer is 3.** Phenylpropanolamine is used to treat urinary incontinence. Dopamine, choice 1, is used to treat shock. Terbutaline, choice 2, is used for bronchodilation. Epinephrine, choice 4, is used to stimulate the heart. Therefore, choices 1, 2, and 4 are incorrect.

112. **The correct answer is 1.** Your clinic should take a blood sample to test for antifreeze poisoning. Choice 2 is incorrect because whole blood is better than serum for testing for antifreeze. Choices 3 and 4 are incorrect because blood will show signs of poisoning before urine or hair.

113. **The correct answer is 4.** Cocker spaniels are predisposed to seborrhea oleosa, which is greasy skin with diffuse scaling, erythema, alopecia,

and inflammation. German shepherds, pugs, and dalmatians are not predisposed to this condition, so choices 1, 2, or 3 are incorrect.

114. **The correct answer is 2.** If a sterile item touches a nonsterile item, it has become nonsterile and should be discarded. Choices 1, 3, and 4 are all incorrect because once an item is no longer sterile, it should not be reused or put on a tray with other items.

115. **The correct answer is 3.** Observing mucus membrane color would be one method used to monitor the oxygenation of a patient under anesthesia. Auscultation of breath sounds, observing the chest wall, and capnography should be used to monitor the patient's respiration, so choices 1, 2, and 4 are incorrect.

116. **The correct answer is 4.** Doberman pinschers are frequently sensitive to the cardiovascular drug digoxin. Great danes, golden retrievers, and Irish setters are not normally sensitive to this medication, so choices 1, 2, and 3 are incorrect.

117. **The correct answer is 4.** You would most likely freeze it, so choice 4 is correct. Urine samples generally can be frozen without harming the results of future testing. Since the urine will be sent to a laboratory, freezing it can help ensure its stability. Choice 1 is incorrect because diluting the urine sample could change some of the test results. Heating the sample, choice 2, is incorrect because urine should not be heated before it is tested. Choice 3 is incorrect because blood samples, not urine samples, should be centrifuged.

118. **The correct answer is 2.** A bone curette is sometimes used to scrape out osteochondritis dissecans lesions. Choice 1, an osteotome, is used to cut through bone. Choice 3, a bone rasp, is used to smooth out any rough bone edges. Choice 4, a rongeur, is used to break up and remove bone. So, choices 1, 3, and 4 are incorrect.

119. **The correct answer is 4.** The veterinary technician does not determine a patient's vital signs while he or she assesses the patient's medical history. Vital signs are determined during the patient's physical examination. Choices 1, 2, and 3 are incorrect because a technician should ask whether the patient's vaccinations are updated, determine the status of the patient's health, and ask about adverse reactions to drugs while assessing the patient's medication history.

120. **The correct answer is 1.** The patient's laboratory test results will most likely show the patient's urea nitrogen levels have increased. High-protein diets cause the protein urea to increase in the body. Choices 2, 3, and 4 are incorrect because bile concentrations, acid concentrations, and ALT levels all increase when a patient is on a low-protein, not a high-protein, diet.

121. **The correct answer is 4.** Sevoflurane requires an agent specific out-of-circle precision vaporizer because of its high vapor pressure and volatility. Choice 1, desflurane, requires an electrically heated vaporizer. Choices 2 and 3, isoflurane and halothane, both require out-of-circle precision vaporizers. With these anesthetics, however, the vaporizer does not need to be agent specific. Therefore, choices 1, 2, and 3 are incorrect.

122. **The correct answer is 2.** Perineal urethrostomy does not require any hair removal during patient preparation. For this procedure, the only requirement is securing the tail to the top of the patient's body. Both feline and canine castrations, choices 1 and 3, require hair removal from the scrotal area. Laparotomy, choice 4, is a type of surgery that includes procedures like splenectomy and ovariohysterectomy. These procedures require extensive hair removal in the affected areas.

123. **The correct answer is 3.** A centrifuge's speed is measured in gravitational forces, or g forces. As the centrifuge spins, it creates a relative centrifugal force (RCF). A centrifuge's acceleration is 981 cm/second/second. Choices 1, 2, and 4 are incorrect because these choices don't represent the speed of a centrifuge or gravity.

124. **The correct answer is 2.** Opioid analgesics relieve pain by blocking the brain's pain impulses. Corticosteroids reduce inflammation, so choice 1 is incorrect. Local anesthetics produce local anesthesia, so choice 3 is not correct. NSAIDs block prostaglandin production, so choice 4 is incorrect.

125. **The correct answer is 4.** Operating room personnel who have been chronically exposed

to nitrous oxide may be at increased risk of a myeloneuropathy. Choices 1 and 3 are incorrect because hepatotoxicity and renal dysfunction can result from excessive exposure to halothane and methoxyflurane, not nitrous oxide. Choice 2 is incorrect because liver damage can be a result of exposure to methoxyflurane.

126. **The correct answer is 4.** Euthanasia by intraperitoneal injection is performed only on very small animals weighing less than 7 kilograms. The methods in choices 1, 2, and 3 are incorrect because they can be used on animals of various sizes.

127. **The correct answer is 2.** Holding the transducer in one place and titling it from side to side describes fanning, so choice 2 is correct. Choice 1, keeping the transducer in one place and applying pressure to the front or the back, describes rocking. Choice 3, holding the transducer in an upright position and moving in different directions, describes sliding. Choice 4, keeping the transducer in contact with skin while pivoting it 90°, describes rotating.

128. **The correct answer is 2.** Different screenings are appropriate for different ailments or symptoms. If an animal is having spinal problems, a radiography screening is the best test to conduct because it will tell the medical team about the condition of the animal's spine and the surrounding bones and tendons. Choices 1 and 3 are incorrect because the medical team will most likely want to know more about the spine before they test the animal's blood or stool. Choice 4 is not correct because the medical team has no evidence to support conducting a biopsy.

129. **The correct answer is 3.** Radiography screenings are sensitive to movement. When a dog pants, its entire body moves and shifts; therefore, the dog's panting may move the animal's body and compromise the results. Choice 1 is incorrect because it is unlikely the dog's panting would fog the screen. Choices 2 and 4 are incorrect because a radiography screening would not be compromised because members of the medical team got annoyed.

130. **The correct answer is 3.** During radiography screenings, it's important to keep patients as still as possible. The results of radiography screenings are best when animals are calm and still, so radiographers most often use anesthetics for restraint. Although anesthetics are used for anesthesia (choice 1), euthanasia (choice 2), and seizure control (choice 4), these choices are incorrect because they are not likely reasons radiographers would use anesthetics.

131. **The correct answer is 2.** Even small amounts of white light can make undeveloped radiographic images slightly foggy. Choices 1 and 3 are incorrect because small amounts of light will not make the entire image black or white. Choice 4 is not correct because light will make the image less clear, not clearer.

132. **The correct answer is 1.** An animal in dorsal recumbency is lying on its back. Choice 2 is incorrect because an animal in right lateral recumbency is on its right side. Choice 3 is not correct because an animal in left lateral recumbency is on its left side. Choice 4 is incorrect because an animal in sternal recumbency is lying on its stomach.

133. **The correct answer is 1.** Buprenorphine is the most potent opioid. This is effective for 8 to 12 hours. Choices 2, 3, and 4 are incorrect because those opioids are less potent than buprenorphine. Meperidine (choice 2) is effective for 1 to 2 hours. Morphine (choice 3) is effective for about 4 hours. Fentanyl (choice 4) is effective for 15 to 30 minutes.

134. **The correct answer is 1.** Autoclaving is the preferred sterilization method because it is fast and effective and because it works on many different materials. Choices 2, 3, and 4 are incorrect because they are not the preferred methods of sterilization. Chemical sterilization (choice 2) takes a long time and may not kill all spores. Boiling (choice 3) is not preferred because it is not always effective and can rust metal instruments. Choice 4, dry heat, is not preferred because this method takes a long time and does not work for materials such as plastic.

135. **The correct answer is 1.** Before you wash or disinfect the skin, you should clip most of the fur from the skin, so choice 1 is correct. Choices 2, 3, and 4 are incorrect because you should disinfect with iodine (choice 2), wash with soap and water (choice 3), and disinfect with alcohol (choice 4) after you clip the fur.

136. **The correct answer is 4.** Epidural anesthesia is most effective on a tail amputation because the

epidural blocks pain on the lower portion of the body, including the tail. Choice 1, 2, and 3 are incorrect because epidural anesthesia would not be effective on the eyes (choice 1), the mouth (choice 2), or the throat (choice 3).

137. **The correct answer is 4.** Vitamin A deficiency does not cause coagulation problems for animals. Animals with vitamin A deficiencies can experience other symptoms such as infection, joint pain, and reproductive problems. Hemophilia (choice 1) is incorrect because it is a genetic disorder that causes coagulation problems. Choices 2 and 3 (liver disease and vitamin K deficiency) are incorrect because they are acquired disorders that are associated with coagulation problems.

138. **The correct answer is 2.** When small animals lose 15–20% of their blood, they begin to experience symptoms of acute blood loss. Choice 1 is not correct because 5–10% is too little blood loss to produce symptoms. Choice 3 is incorrect because at 35–40% blood loss, small animals typically experience hemorrhagic shock. Choice 4 is incorrect because animals with a blood loss of more than 40% have already experienced hemorrhagic shock.

139. **The correct answer is 1.** When you underfill the tube, the ratio of EDTA to blood is too high. The high amount of EDTA causes the erythrocytes (red blood cells) to shrink. When the erythrocytes shrink, the sample could have a decreased packed cell volume, so choice 1 is correct. Choice 2 is incorrect because heparin tubes, not EDTA tubes, can cause poorly stained leukocytes (white blood cells). Choice 3 is incorrect because sodium heparin tubes can show a false increase in sodium levels. Choice 4 is incorrect because heparin plasma can be unreliable for measuring bile and acid levels.

140. **The correct answer is 4.** Pilocarpine, which is a miotic, is used to constrict the pupil. Tetracaine, choice 1, is an ophthalmic anesthetic. Atropine, choice 2, is a mydriatic used to dilate the pupil. Cyclosporine, choice 3, increases tear production.

141. **The correct answer is 1.** Furosemide can be administered intramuscularly, as well as intravenously or orally. Spironolactone and chlorothiazide, choices 2 and 3, can be administered only orally. Mannitol, choice 4, can only be administered via intravenous infusion.

142. **The correct answer is 2.** The tank yoke connectors are a common site of leaks in high-pressure anesthetic machines. Unidirectional valves, the pop-off valve, and the soda lime canister, choices 1, 3, and 4, are all common leak sites in low-pressure anesthetic machines.

143. **The correct answer is 2.** Prostaglandins are administered to lyse the corpus luteum. Estrogens are used to prevent pregnancy after mismating, so choice 1 is incorrect. Progestins are used to return a mare in transitional anestrus to proestrus, so choice 3 is not correct. Oxytocin is used to induce uterine contractions, so choice 4 is not correct.

144. **The correct answer is 3.** The Bain system breathing circuit is most useful with patients undergoing procedures involving the head. The Bain system uses less tubing than other breathing circuits and is less obstructive during head procedures. The Bain system would not be particularly useful for procedures involving the legs, chest, or spine, so choices 1, 2, and 4 are incorrect.

145. **The correct answer is 4.** Methoxyflurane is no longer commonly used because of its potential severe side effects. Methoxyflurane can lead to kidney or liver impairment or birth defects. Sevoflurane, halothane, and isoflurane, choices 1, 2, and 3, are all used commonly today.

146. **The correct answer is 2.** Amitraz cannot be administered to cats because of potential toxicity. This medication, which is designed to eradicate Demodex mites and other ectoparasites, can be very toxic to cats and may lead to death. Selamectin, imidacloprid, and nitenpyram are all safe to use with cats, so choices 1, 3, and 4 are incorrect.

147. **The correct answer is 1.** Anesthesia depth can be difficult to control with non-precision vaporizers. Precision vaporizers compensate for temperature and back-pressure, are generally very expensive, and must be serviced every six to twelve months, so choices 2, 3, and 4 are incorrect.

148. **The correct answer is 4.** Nitrous oxide is nonirritative and sweet smelling. Choice 1 can refer to either sevoflurane or desflurane. Choice 2 refers to desflurane. Choice 3 refers to halothane.

149. **The correct answer is 3.** Dimercaprol can be used to treat a patient suffering from mercury toxicity. This medication is also used to treat gold, arsenic, and lead toxicity. Antivenin polyvalent is used to treat poisonous snake envenomation, so choice 1 is incorrect. Naloxone is used to treat opioid agonist reversal, so choice 2 is incorrect. Cyproheptadine is used to treat serotonin syndrome, so choice 4 is incorrect.

150. **The correct answer is 2.** Phenobarbital is most often used as a sedative for excitable dogs. Pentobarbital, methohexital, and thiopental—choices 1, 3, and 4—are not commonly used for this purpose.

151. **The correct answer is 2.** Mibolerone, an androgen, is used to treat pseudocyesis, or false pregnancy, in adult dogs. Oxytocin, choice 1, is used to induce labor. Desmopressin, choice 3, is used to control diabetes insipidus. Medroxy-progesterone, choice 4, is used to treat various behavioral and dermatological conditions.

152. **The correct answer is 4.** Etomidate may cause phlebitis upon injection, particularly in small veins. Propofol supports bacterial growth due to soy content, so choice 1 is incorrect. Guaifenesin exists in a powder form and is reconstituted with water or dextrose, so choice 2 in incorrect. Fentanyl is referred to as a neuroleptanalgesic, so choice 3 is incorrect.

153. **The correct answer is 3.** Griseofulvin is a known teratogen in cats, meaning that it can cause birth defects or spontaneous abortion in feline patients. Nystatin, fluconazole, and terbinafine are not known teratogens, so choices 1, 2, and 4 are incorrect.

154. **The correct answer is 4.** The medical team has 4 to 6 hours to clean and close an open surgical wound before infection becomes likely. Choices 1, 2, and 3 are incorrect because surgical teams have more time to close surgical wounds than these choices indicate.

155. **The correct answer is 4.** Silk is a nonabsorbable suture material that may act like a wick and allow migration of contamination. Choices 1, 2, and 3, polypropylene, stainless steel, and nylon, will not act as wicks and allow the migration of contamination.

156. **The correct answer is 2.** Patients with respiratory problems that affect their ability to oxygenate should not be anesthetized with nitrous oxide. Use of nitrous oxide in such a patient significantly increases the risk of hypoxia. Choices 1, 3, and 4 (halothane, sevoflurane, and isoflurane) are all safer to use under these circumstances.

157. **The correct answer is 1.** H2 blockers are systemic antacids designed to prevent the production of hydrochloric acid. Misoprostol blocks the release of hydrogen ions and stimulates mucus and bicarbonate in the stomach, so choice 2 is incorrect. Omeprazole prevents the pumping of hydrogen ions into the stomach, so choice 3 is not correct. Nonsystemic antacids, such as Maalox or Mylanta, neutralize acid that is already present in the stomach, so choice 4 is not correct.

158. **The correct answer is 3.** The presence of puss does not indicate inflammation of a wound or surgical site, so choice 3 is correct. The loss of function of an area (choice 1), swelling (choice 2), and redness (choice 4) are all symptoms of inflammation. Other symptoms of inflammation include heat and pain.

159. **The correct answer is 3.** Diltiazem is a calcium channel blocker. Isoproterenol (choice 1) is an adrenergic. Pimobendan (choice 2) is an inodilator. Captopril (choice 4) is an ACE inhibitor.

160. **The correct answer is 3.** When clipping an animal prior to surgery on an open wound, water-soluble lubricant should be placed in the wound in order to prevent contamination from loose hair. At this point, water-soluble lubricant would not be used to decontaminate the wound, encourage faster healing, or to clear the wound of dried or excess blood, so choices 1, 2, and 4 are incorrect.

161. **The correct answer is 3.** Mixing different metals in the same ultrasonic cleaning cycle may result in corrosion. Spotting, pitting, and staining may result if surgical instruments are not properly cleaned after use, but they are not common side effects of ultrasonic cleaning. Therefore, choices 1, 2, and 4 are incorrect.

162. **The correct answer is 4.** Metzenbaum scissors have pointed or blunt tips with straight or curved blades. Mayo scissors have blunt tips with straight or curved blades, so choice 1 is incorrect. Wire-cutting scissors have short, thick jaws with serrated edges, so choice 2 is incorrect. Littauer and Spencer suture removal scissors have blunt tips with one blade terminating into a thin, curved hook, so choice 3 is incorrect.

163. **The correct answer is 4.** Hemostatic forceps are used during surgical procedures to ligate blood vessels or tissues. Halsted mosquito forceps are used to control capillary bleeding, so choice 1 is incorrect. Choices 2 and 3, Rochester-Pean forceps and Rochester-Carmalt forceps, are used to clamp large bundles of tissues that contain blood vessels, so those choices are also incorrect.

164. **The correct answer is 1.** When an animal is anesthetized prior to an orogastric intubation, the use of a cuffed, tight-fitting endotracheal tube is indicated because this method will prevent aspiration of the administered material. Choices 2, 3, and 4 are incorrect because the tube is not better tolerated than others, the changes of the tube being disrupted are not reduced, and the tube does not ensure a shorter procedure time.

165. **The correct answer is 3.** Schirmer's tear test can be used to diagnose keratoconjunctivitis siccca, otherwise known as dry eye. This test would not be diagnostic for conjunctivitis, glaucoma, or cherry eye, choices 1, 2, and 4.

166. **The correct answer is 2.** Neutrophils and monocytes travel to the site of a wound to remove foreign material, necrotic tissue, and bacteria in the debridement phase of wound healing. The inflammatory phase, choice 1, is the first phase and includes the initial clotting and scabbing of the wound. The repair phase, choice 3, follows debridement and includes the production of collagen and granulation tissue. The maturation phase, choice 4, is the final stage in wound healing and involves the remodeling of collagen fibers and fibrous tissues.

167. **The correct answer is 2.** When maintaining hemostasis for the surgeon, you should dab, not wipe, the area with a gauze square, so choice 2 is correct. Placing the suction tip near the tissue

(choice 1), rather than directly on the tissue, is correct procedure. It would be appropriate to count the number of used and discarded gauze squares, so choice 3 is incorrect. As a surgical assistant, you may cut suture material after the suture has been properly placed, so choice 4 is also incorrect.

168. **The correct answer is 3.** Surgical instruments should always be washed with a neutral pH cleanser. Neutral pH cleansers are effective for cleaning and safe to use on stainless steel. Chlorhexidine, surgical scrub, or dish soap (choices 1, 2, and 4) should never be used on surgical instruments because their high chlorine contents can cause spotting and corrosion.

169. **The correct answer is 3.** You should exercise special care when applying isopropyl alcohol to a Chihuahua because this substance can cause serious complications in small animals that may have difficulty maintaining proper body temperature. None of the breeds in choices 1, 2, or 4 would be likely to experience temperature control problems with exposure to isopropyl alcohol.

170. **The correct answer is 2.** Non-fresh surgical milk may cause contamination of surgical instruments. Non-fresh surgical milk may contain bacterial growth that can contaminate surgical instruments. Non-fresh surgical milk would not cause staining or corrosion, decreased lubrication, or spotting, so choices 1, 3, and 4 are incorrect.

171. **The correct answer is 2.** Tapered point suture needles are most commonly used on muscle. The soft tissue of muscles is usually more susceptible to tearing or other damage, so tapered point suture needles are used to reduce the incidence of trauma as much as possible. Skin, tendons, and cartilage (choices 1, 3, and 4) are tougher tissues that generally require cutting point suture needles.

172. **The correct answer is 3.** Allis tissue forceps are an example of self-retaining forceps. This means that these forceps have a ratchet-locking device that grasps and retracts tissue. Russian tissue forceps, dressing forceps, and Adson forceps, choices 1, 2, and 4, are all examples of thumb forceps.

173. **The correct answer is 3.** The veterinarian's instructions mean: Give the patient eye drops in both eyes twice per day. The abbreviation O.U.

means in "both eyes," and the abbreviation b.i.d. means "twice per day." Choices 1, 2, and 4 are incorrect because the abbreviation meaning "right eye" is O.D., and the abbreviation meaning "once per day" is s.i.d.

174. The correct answer is 3. A dog that ingested a full bottle of its owner's medication should be given emetics to empty its stomach contents, so choice 3 is correct. Choice 1 is incorrect because unconscious animals should never be given emetics. Choice 2 is not correct because emetics should not be administered when the animal ingested a corrosive toxin. Choice 4 is incorrect because rabbits should never be given emetics.

175. The correct answer is 3. Horses with broken femurs are put into the "dead, dying, or euthanized" category during triage. Horses need to stand because they have circulation problems when they lie down, and they need all four legs to stand properly. So, horses with broken femurs must be euthanized. Choices 1, 2, and 4 are incorrect because dogs, cats, and rabbits with broken femurs can generally be treated with bandages, surgery, or similar therapies.

176. The correct answer is 2. Injections administered below the top layers of skin are subcutaneous, so choice 2 is correct. Choice 1 is incorrect because intramuscular injections are administered directly into the muscle. Intravenous injections are administered into veins, so choice 3 is not correct. Choice 4 is incorrect because gastrointestinal means relating to the stomach and intestine and does not describe a route of injection administration.

177. The correct answer is 3. A laceration is a wound that includes major damage to the skin and other soft tissue and easily gets infected. An abrasion is a wound that is characterized by the exposure of the dermis and is usually not serious, so choice 1 is incorrect. Choice 2 is not correct because a puncture wound, not a laceration, is one that does not show obvious signs on the skin's surface, but goes deep into the tissue. Choice 4 is incorrect because a hematoma involves the rupture of a blood vessel below the skin's surface, where blood pools.

178. The correct answer is 4. Recumbent patients often cannot groom or clean themselves so you should clean and groom the patient on a daily basis. Grooming is also important for recumbent patients because they get bored easily, and they enjoy the attention. Choice 1 is incorrect because recumbent patients should stay in kennels large enough to lie in, but not large enough to move around in. Choice 2 is not correct because recumbent patients get bored quickly, so keeping them in an area with a lot of activity can keep them stimulated. Choice 3 is incorrect because recumbent patients need padded, soft bedding to keep them comfortable.

179. The correct answer is 3. A metal comb is the best grooming tool to remove mats from animals' coats, so choice 3 is correct. Choice 1 is incorrect because double-sided brushes work best for grooming silky coats. Choice 2 is not correct because sticker brushes work best for pulling out loose hair. Choice 4 is incorrect because hound gloves work best for routine grooming.

180. The correct answer is 1. A dog weighing 10 pounds would weigh 4.53 kilograms when measured metrically. Choices 2, 3, and 4 are all incorrect.

181. The correct answer is 2. A patient would most likely be immobilized by its bandages to stop the patient from moving a fractured limb. Patients could make the damage of a fractured limb worse by moving it, so immobilizing the limb is a good idea. Choices 1, 3, and 4 are incorrect because immobilizing a patient will not stop hemorrhaging (choice 1), prevent infection (choice 3), or reduce swelling (choice 4).

182. The correct answer is 2. In a simple fracture, the bone is broken into two pieces. Choice 1 is incorrect because a complicated fracture occurs when the broken bone damages organs or vessels. A compound fracture occurs when the broken bone causes a wound on the skin, so choice 3 is incorrect. Choice 4 is not correct because a multiple fracture occurs when the bone is broken into more than two pieces.

183. The correct answer is 2. Fluid therapy is contraindicated in the event of pulmonary contusions because these contusions may cause fluid to shift into the lungs, which can lead to pulmonary edema. Choice 1, although not likely to suggest the need for fluid therapy, would not be a contraindication. Choices 3 and 4 are both common signs of dehydration and would indicate the need for fluid therapy.

184. The correct answer is 2. A progressive lengthening of the PR interval on successive beats accompanied by the occurrence of P waves without QRS complexes would indicate Type I second-degree AV block. Choice 1 is indicated by an abnormally long PR interval. Choice 3 is indicated by a PR interval of generally normal duration with random dropped beats. Choice 4 is indicated by a lack of relationship between P waves and QRS complexes.

185. The correct answer is 1. A Schirmer's tear test result of 9 millimeters of moisture would indicate keratitis sicca in a feline patient. Keratitis sicca is indicated in cats with less than 10 millimeters of moisture. Choices 2, 3, and 4 could indicate keratoconjunctivitis in canine, not feline, patients.

186. The correct answer is 4. A Robert Jones bandage, which is made of several layers of tightly compressed rolled cotton, is used to stabilize a fracture before surgery. Choice 1 is used to support the hind limb following reduction of hip luxation. Choice 2 is used to prevent excessive abduction of hind limbs. Choice 3 is used to provide shoulder support following surgery.

187. The correct answer is 3. Testosterone is an anabolic steroid and a controlled substance. As a result, veterinary technicians are required to store this drug in a secure location. None of the drugs listed in choices 1, 2, or 4 are controlled substances and do not require secure storage.

188. The correct answer is 3. Chondrosarcoma is a malignant tumor of cartilage. A tumor of bone, choice 1, is called osteosarcoma. A tumor of fibrous tissue, choice 2, is called fibrosarcoma. A tumor of blood vessels, choice 4, is called hemangiosarcoma.

189. The correct answer is 3. Hyperthyroidism is a possible cause of sinus tachycardia because excessive amounts of thyroid hormone increase the heart's force of contraction and its demand for oxygen. Acidosis, hypokalemia, and ventricular concentric hypertrophy (choices 1, 2, and 4) are all potential causes of premature ventricular contraction.

190. The correct answer is 4. A fluid-filled blister measuring 0.3 centimeter would be called a vesicle. A bulla, choice 1, is the same as a vesicle, except that it measures more than 0.5 centimeter. A wheal, choice 2, also known as a hive, is a flat-topped, raised area of skin that is noticeably redder or paler than the surrounding area. A papule, choice 3, is a circular, reddened area of elevated skin.

191. The correct answer is 3. Povidone-iodine solution is inactivated by exudates, blood, and organic material, so its effects will last only a few hours. Choice 1 describes chlorhexidine diacetate solution, which has a longer lasting effect because it is not inactivated by organic material. Choices 2 and 4 both describe hydrogen peroxide.

192. The correct answer is 4. When performing venipuncture through the jugular vein, the patient should be placed in sternal recumbency, or on its stomach. With the patient in this position, the restrainer can hold the animal's front legs with one hand and raise its head with the other, exposing the jugular vein. Patients are not normally placed in left or right lateral recumbency (choices 1 and 3) or dorsal recumbency (choice 2) for this procedure.

193. The correct answer is 2. When performing venipuncture, you can ensure adequate blood flow by occluding the vein. Occluding the vein prevents blood from flowing back to the heart and allows it to accumulate in the vein. Applying alcohol to the puncture site (choice 1) will clean the area and help the venipuncturist to find the vein before inserting the needle. Inserting the needle with the bevel facing downwards (choice 3) would inhibit blood flow. Pulling back the plunger as quickly as possible (choice 4) could interfere with both the collection process and the sample itself.

194. The correct answer is 3. All types of samples should be tested as soon as possible after they're collected, so it's important to have the owner bring in the sample as soon as possible after it's taken. Choice 1 is incorrect because urine samples should be collected right after the animal wakes up, not right before it goes to sleep. Choice 2 is not correct because when the owner collects the sample, he or she should wait a few seconds to begin to collect the urine, as the first part of the sample could contain bacteria that could change some test results. Choice 4 is not correct because the owner should collect the sample right after the animal wakes up, as giving the animal food and water could change certain levels in the urine.

195. **The correct answer is 2.** This patient's condition is referred to as a caudal crossbite. A rostral crossbite (choice 1) occurs when one or more of the maxillary incisors are displaced so as to have become lingual to mandibular incisors. A distoclusion (choice 3) occurs when the teeth in the mandible are distal to their maxillary equivalents. A mesioclusion (choice 4) occurs when the mandibular teeth occlude mesial to their maxillary counterparts.

196. **The correct answer is 2.** A 10% change in a patient's white blood cell count from one day to the next is most likely insignificant because a 10% change is too low to cause concern. A 10% change in white blood cell counts could be due to slight changes in procedure in the lab, so it is not generally considered significant. Choice 1 is incorrect because changes between 10–20% are usually due to laboratory procedures, rather than changes in the patient's blood. Choice 3 is not correct because slight changes in white blood cell counts are usually not significant. Choice 4 is incorrect because white blood cell counts are important for determining a patient's health, and big changes in the count could be a sign of a health problem.

197. **The correct answer is 4.** A veterinary technician would most likely perform a CRT test to check for heart disease. To conduct the test, the technician will press on the patient's gums to see how quickly the capillaries in the gums refill with blood. Since slow blood flow could indicate heart problems, this test can help diagnose heart disease. Choices 1, 2, and 3 are incorrect because blood flow speed is generally not helpful for diagnosing cancer (choice 1), liver disease (choice 2), or cataracts (choice 3).

198. **The correct answer is 2.** Sodium and potassium are generally analyzed together during a chemical panel, so choice 2 is correct. Choices 1, 3, and 4 are incorrect because although cholesterol, calcium, and serum glutamic pyruvic transaminase (SGPT) levels may be checked during a chemical panel, they are not analyzed with the potassium levels.

199. **The correct answer is 4.** The paper covered in urine from a cat infected with ear mites would be disposed of in the regular waste, rather than the biomedical waste. Choices 1, 2, and 3 are incorrect because those items should be disposed of in the biomedical waste. The needle (choice 1) and the scalpel (choice 3) must be disposed of in the biomedical waste because they have sharp edges. The rubbing tubing (choice 2) must be disposed of in the biomedical waste because the animal is infected with a disease that can be transmitted to humans.

200. **The correct answer is 1.** Incisors are used primarily for cutting and nibbling. Canines (choice 2) are primarily used for holding and tearing. Premolars (choice 3) are primarily used for cutting, shearing, and holding. Molars (choice 4) are primarily used for grinding.

PART III

Types of Questions on the Veterinary Technician National Exam (VTNE)

CHAPTER 4

Pharmacy and Pharmacology Questions

OVERVIEW

- Preparing for pharmacy and pharmacology questions
- Tips for answering pharmacy and pharmacology questions
- Practice questions
- Answer key and explanations
- Summing it up

PREPARING FOR PHARMACY AND PHARMACOLOGY QUESTIONS

Pharmacy and pharmacology questions are one type of question on the VTNE. This group of questions makes up 14 percent (28 items) of the exam. The questions pertaining to pharmacy and pharmacology test your knowledge of the wide variety of drugs used in veterinary medicine and your ability to use them properly.

Pharmacology, which is the science of the origin, nature, chemistry, effects, and applications of drugs, is a very significant part of a veterinary technician's job. Although veterinary technicians are not allowed to prescribe drugs themselves, they may be responsible for filling prescriptions, dispensing drugs, or administering drugs. As a result, it is important that any prospective veterinary technician have a solid understanding of the wide variety of drugs used in veterinary medicine.

Pharmacy and pharmacology questions ask about preparing, administering, and dispensing drugs prescribed to patients, as well as educating clients about the drugs being administered to or dispensed for their pets.

Some questions may ask you to identify the classification of a drug, the generic or trade name of a drug, the functions of a drug, the correct drug to use in a given situation, the possible side effects associated with a particular drug, the form a drug comes in, the appropriate routes of administration for particular drugs, the correct dosages of a drug, or the indications and contraindications for dispensing a drug.

When preparing for pharmacy and pharmacology questions, you should make sure you understand pharmacy procedures, pharmacokinetics, administering medications, the legal requirements associated with certain drugs, the dangers presented by potentially hazardous drugs, and the safety precautions you should take when handling them.

The VTNE also includes questions that test your ability to effectively communicate with clients about their pet's health and pharmacological needs. These questions may deal with prescription instructions, special orders from the veterinarian, explaining the function of a drug to the client, and more.

The multiple-choice questions on the VTNE may require you to choose the correct answer from a series of four possible choices, identify the most accurate statement, identify the least accurate statement, or correctly complete an incomplete statement.

The pharmacy and pharmacology domain of the VTNE includes questions based on many different topics such as:

- Drug classifications

- Toxicology

- Routes of administration

- Contraindications and side effects

- Normal and abnormal drug reactions and drug interactions

- Legal requirements and procedures for preparing, storing, and dispensing pharmacological and biological agents

- Applied mathematics

- Common animal diseases

- Preanesthetic, anesthetic, and analgesic medications

- Techniques for communicating with the veterinary team and clients

TIPS FOR ANSWERING PHARMACY AND PHARMACOLOGY QUESTIONS

Remember these hints when answering pharmacy and pharmacology questions on the VTNE:

1. **A drug can have different effects on different animals.** A drug that has a particular effect on one type of animal may have a very different effect on another. Some animals can have unique reactions to certain medications that may range from simple ineffectiveness to mild or moderate irritation or even severe toxicity and death. When you are answering pharmacy and pharmacology questions on the VTNE, pay close attention to species, breeds, ages, sizes, and medical conditions of the animals in the questions. All these factors will help you determine the right drugs and dosages for the animals.

2. **Some drugs may have more than one application.** Not all drugs serve only a single purpose. Some drugs can effectively treat a variety of conditions that affect different body systems. In some cases, you may need to be aware of alternative uses for particular drugs. Also, be aware that the same drug could be used in two different ways because of the particular animals it is being used on.

3. **Remember when you should or should not use a particular drug.** Every situation is different. When you are asked to identify the correct treatment for a patient's condition, remember to pay close attention to all of the patient's signs and symptoms. Certain symptoms may indicate or contraindicate the use of a particular drug. Make sure that the drug you choose is right for the intended patient.

DRUG CLASSIFICATIONS

Antimicrobials

Analgesics and anti-inflammatory drugs

Anesthetics and other central nervous
  system drugs

Cardiovascular drugs

Respiratory drugs

Gastrointestinal drugs

Antiparasitic drugs

Hormones and other endocrine drugs

Chemotherapeutic and immunological agents

Antidotes and reversal agents

Topical drugs

PRACTICE QUESTIONS

1. Which of the following is a corticosteroid?
   1. Hyaluronate
   2. Butorphanol
   3. Triamcinolone
   4. Piroxicam

2. Which type of adrenergic drug is used to treat shock or hypotension?
   1. Terbutaline
   2. Dopamine
   3. Xylazine
   4. Epinephrine

3. You are instructing a patient's owner about administering her pet's new medication at home. The veterinarian's directions indicate that the medication should be given "per os q.i.d." What do these instructions mean?
   1. Intravenously, two times a day
   2. Orally, two times a day
   3. Intravenously, four times a day
   4. Orally, four times a day

4. Florfenicol can be administered either intramuscularly or:
   1. orally.
   2. intravenously.
   3. subcutaneously.
   4. topically.

5. Periactin is the trade name for:
   1. Hydroxyzine.
   2. Cyproheptadine.
   3. Diphenhydramine.
   4. Clemastine.

6. Which of the following cardiovascular drugs is a vasodilator?
   1. Lidocaine
   2. Spironolactone
   3. Prazosin
   4. Benazepril

7. Which antiparasitic drug can be used to treat hookworm?
   1. Pyrantel
   2. Epsiprantel
   3. Piperazine
   4. Praziquantel

8. Idoxuridine is administered:
   1. orally.
   2. intramuscularly.
   3. topically.
   4. intravenously.

9. Which type of laxative helps relieve constipation by increasing stool water content and stimulating peristalsis in the gastrointestinal tract?
   1. Lubricants
   2. Bulk-producing agents
   3. Hyperosmotics
   4. Stool softeners

10. Which of the following respiratory drugs is a decongestant?
    1. Doxapram
    2. Hydrocodone
    3. Acetylcysteine
    4. Phenylpropanolamine

ANSWER KEY AND EXPLANATIONS

1. 3	3. 4	5. 2	7. 1	9. 2
2. 2	4. 3	6. 3	8. 3	10. 4

1. **The correct answer is 3.** Triamcinolone is a corticosteroid. Hyaluronate, choice 1, is a glycosaminoglycan. Butorphanol, choice 2, is a muscle relaxant. Piroxicam, choice 4, is an NSAID.

2. **The correct answer is 2.** Dopamine is an adrenergic drug used to treat shock or hypotension. Terbutaline, choice 1, is used for bronchodilation. Xylazine, choice 3, is used as an analgesic or sedative. Epinephrine, choice 4, is used to stimulate the heart.

3. **The correct answer is 4.** The veterinarian's instructions mean that the medication should be administered orally, four times a day. Choice 1 would be written as "IV b.i.d." Choice 2 would be written as "per os b.i.d." Choice 3 would be written as "IV q.i.d."

4. **The correct answer is 3.** Florfenicol can be administered either intramuscularly or subcutaneously. This antimicrobial medication cannot be administered orally (choice 1), intravenously (choice 2), or topically (choice 4).

5. **The correct answer is 2.** Periactin is the trade name for cyproheptadine. Atarax is the trade name for hydroxyzine (choice 1). Benadryl is the trade name for diphenhydramine (choice 3). Tavist is the trade name for clemastine (choice 4).

6. **The correct answer is 3.** Prazosin is a type of cardiovascular drug known as a vasodilator. Lidocaine (choice 1) is an antiarrhythmic. Spironolactone (choice 2) is a diuretic. Benazepril (choice 4) is an ACE inhibitor.

7. **The correct answer is 1.** Pyrantel is an antiparasitic drug that can be used to treat hookworm. It can also be used to treat roundworm. Epsiprantel and praziquantel, choices 2 and 4, can be used to treat tapeworms. Piperazine, choice 3, can be used to treat roundworm.

8. **The correct answer is 3.** Idoxuridine is administered topically. Idoxuridine is an antiviral drug used to treat feline herpes infections. Choices 1, 2, and 4 are all incorrect administration routes for idoxuridine.

9. **The correct answer is 2.** Bulk-producing agents help relieve constipation by increasing stool water content and stimulating peristalsis in the gastrointestinal tract. Lubricants, choice 1, can be used to help make passing stool easier. Hyperosmotics, choice 3, work by drawing water into the bowels which softens the stool. Stool softeners, choice 4, allow water to penetrate the contents of the gastrointestinal tract.

10. **The correct answer is 4.** Phenylpropanolamine is a decongestant. Doxapram, choice 1, is a stimulant. Hydrocodone, choice 2, is an antitussive. Acetylcysteine, choice 3, is a mucolytic.

SUMMING IT UP

- Pharmacy and pharmacology questions will require an understanding of pharmacy procedures, pharmacokinetics, drug classifications, the uses and effects of drugs, administration routes and techniques, and proper ways to communicate with clients about their pets' medications.

- When studying for questions pertaining to preparing, administering, and dispensing drugs prescribed to patients, remember to focus on drug dosages, intended effects, side effects, administration routes, and so on. You will need to know as much about the drugs used in veterinary medicine as possible.

- Pay close attention to specific details in the questions. The species, breed, age, size, and medical condition can determine which drugs and dosages particular animals should receive. You may choose the wrong drug or dose if you do not know all the details. Also, remember that some drugs have multiple purposes and are used differently in different situations. Some drugs should not be used in specific circumstances.

- When you prepare for questions associated with client education, be sure that you know enough about the drugs you will be working with to be able to keep your clients properly informed about the medications being prescribed for their pets, especially if they will be expected to administer the drugs themselves. Be sure that you can explain the veterinarian's orders in a way that is easy for clients to understand.

CHAPTER 5

Surgical Preparation and Assisting Questions

OVERVIEW

- **Preparing for surgical preparation and assisting questions**
- **Tips for answering surgical preparation and assisting questions**
- **Practice questions**
- **Answer key and explanations**
- **Summing it up**

PREPARING FOR SURGICAL PREPARATION AND ASSISTING QUESTIONS

The second group of questions on the VTNE is surgical preparation and assisting questions. This group accounts for 16 percent (32 items) of the questions on the exam. These questions test your knowledge of surgical procedures, preparation and maintenance of the operating room, preparation of patients for surgery, and performing as a sterile or nonsterile assistant during surgical procedures.

The surgical preparation and assisting questions are multiple-choice questions that deal with veterinary technicians' duties before, during, and after surgery. Some of the questions may also ask you to identify the correct name of surgical procedures or surgical tools, based on definitions or scenarios. Other questions may ask you to identify one true statement among three incorrect statements or to determine which of four statements is incorrect or correct.

To correctly answer questions about surgery preparation and assisting, you will need to know the names of surgical procedures, the uses of surgical instruments and equipment, sterilization and disinfectant techniques, and ideal operating room conditions. You may also be asked about suturing techniques, setting up the surgical station, disposing of surgical materials, and fasting procedures for different animals.

Some questions focus on sterilization and other aseptic techniques. You may be asked about using the autoclave and how it works. Questions may also cover proper sterilization techniques of instruments and equipment, the proper ways to sterilize the environment prior to surgery, and ways of maintaining a sterile environment during surgery.

COMMON SURGICAL PROCEDURES

- Amputation
- Bloat surgery
- Bone fracture repair
- Cataract removal
- Cystotomy (bladder)
- Debarking
- Declawing
- Descenting
- Exploratory

- Femoral head ostectomy (hip dysplasia)
- Neuter
- Otoplasty (ear cropping)
- Ovariohysterectomy (spay)
- Tail docking
- Thyroidectomy (removal of thyroid)
- Triple pelvic osteotomy (hip dysplasia)
- Tumor removal
- Wound repair

Surgical preparation and assisting questions are based on a number of different topics including the following:

Anatomy

Animal handling

Aseptic and sterilization techniques for equipment and supplies

Cleaning and disinfecting the surgical area before and after surgery

Common animal diseases

Environmental health and safety procedures

Medical terms

Monitoring the animal during surgery

Patient positioning

Sterile and nonsterile surgical assistance

Surgical procedures

Suturing techniques

To prepare for these questions, focus on studying information related to these topics. Remember, veterinarians treat animals of all shapes and sizes, including cattle, dogs, cats, horses, goats, lizards, rabbits, and so on, so be sure to familiarize yourself with information about as many animals as possible. You should know the most commonly performed surgical procedures and which types of procedures are performed on specific types of animals. You should also review information about what common surgical instruments and equipment look like and how they are used.

TIPS FOR ANSWERING SURGICAL PREPARATION AND ASSISTING QUESTIONS

Remember the following tips when answering surgical preparation and assisting questions on the VTNE:

1. **Not all surgeries are the same.** All animals have different anatomies and, therefore, require different types of surgical procedures. For example, hip dysplasia, which is a common condition in large dog breeds, can be treated with several different surgeries. Different surgeries are performed on dogs based on the animals' ages and sizes. Understanding which procedures are performed on which animals is important. Surgery preparation and assistance may also cover the names of common surgical procedures and the reasons why these surgeries are performed.

2. **Sterilization and aseptic techniques are vital.** The equipment and instruments used during surgical procedures must be sterile. From the operating table to the surgical tools to the technician's hands, everything must be disinfected to prevent the spread of infection. If you drop a piece of equipment on the floor, do you know what to do? These types of questions may ask you how to sterilize an instrument, how long to wash your hands, or what to do

if you drop an instrument on the floor. As long as you know the proper protocols when it comes to sterilization, you should have no problem answering these questions.

3. **Every instrument has its use.** A chef cannot cook a meal without proper kitchen equipment, and a veterinarian cannot perform surgery without the proper instruments. As a surgical assistant, you must know the names and uses of surgical equipment. If the surgeon needs a hemostat, you would not hand him or her a pair of scissors. These types of questions ask you to identify a tool based on a description or by its use.

COMMONLY USED SURGICAL INSTRUMENTS/EQUIPMENT

- Forceps (Adson, Babcock, Kelly, Littlewood, Ochsner, Ruskin)

- Needles

- Needle holders (Mathieu, Mayo-Hegar)

- Scalpels

- Scissors (Carless, Lister, Mayo, Metzenbaum)

- Retractors (Malleable, Volkmann, Weitlaner)

---

4. **Watch the wording of questions.** Some questions contain words such as *except*, *most likely*, *generally*, *usually*, *most commonly*, and so on. When reading questions, be on the lookout for these words so you know exactly what each question is asking. If you read the questions too quickly, you may miss words such as *except*, and you could choose the incorrect answer. Carefully read each question and answer choice before selecting an answer.

PRACTICE QUESTIONS

1. You are packing a surgical pack for an upcoming surgery. You should:
   1. pack swabs and drapes apart from other instruments and tubing.
   2. put the instruments directly onto a metal or plastic instrument tray.
   3. wrap the pack so when it is opened, the outer layers do not cover the stand.
   4. wrap the instruments with a water-resistant cover or drape.

2. Which of the following could worsen the condition of a patient going into shock?
   1. Preventing more blood loss
   2. Applying direct heat to the body
   3. Administering intravenous fluids
   4. Preventing the body from losing heat

3. Which type of scissors would you use to remove bandages from a patient?
   1. Lister
   2. Carless
   3. Mayo
   4. Metzenbaum

4. Chest tubes used for drainage are generally placed between the ribs at the:
   1. first or second intercostal space.
   2. fourth and fifth intercostal space.
   3. seventh or eighth intercostal space.
   4. tenth and eleventh intercostal space.

5. A patient is about to undergo ophthalmological surgery. Which of these preoperative diagnostic aids can help the veterinary team determine damage of a patient's cornea?
   1. Fluorescein staining
   2. Electroretinography
   3. Schirmer tear test
   4. Ultrasonography

6. Which of the following are classified as dissecting forceps?
   1. Littlewood
   2. Adson
   3. Ruskin
   4. Babcock

7. Which of the following statements is true about postoperative procedures?
   1. Dull items, such as swabs, should be removed from the surgical instrument tray first.
   2. Delicate surgical instruments can be cleaned with the rest of the instruments.
   3. Instruments should be cleaned under cool water using abrasive brushes.
   4. Surgical instruments should be cleaned as soon as possible after surgery.

8. Which of the following is an example of using acceptable aseptic technique?
   1. A surgeon asks one of the scrubbed team members to pick up a sterile instrument from the tray.
   2. A nonsterile team member reaches over the patient to move a instrument for the surgeon.
   3. One of the surgery team members turns his back toward the surgical team and the patient.
   4. The instrument table drapes are made from fabric that is not water resistant.

9. A veterinarian schedules an operation for an 8-year-old golden retriever. Before the operation, the golden retriever must fast for:
   1. 1 hour.
   2. 4 hours.
   3. 12 hours.
   4. 15 hours.

10. Which of the following procedures is performed *first* during preparation for limb surgery?
    1. Scrubbing for sterilization
    2. Wrapping the paw or foot
    3. Clipping hair or fur from site
    4. Evacuating bladder contents

ANSWER KEY AND EXPLANATIONS

1. 4	3. 1	5. 1	7. 4	9. 3
2. 2	4. 3	6. 2	8. 1	10. 4

1. **The correct answer is 4.** When assembling a surgical pack, you should wrap the instruments with a water-resistant cover or drape. Choice 1 is incorrect because you should pack swabs and drapes with the other instruments. Choice 2 is incorrect because you should cover the plastic or metal tray with a piece of linen. Choice 3 is incorrect because, ideally, the outer layers of the pack will cover the instrument stand when it is opened.

2. **The correct answer is 2.** Applying direct heat to the body of a patient going into shock could worsen the patient's condition. When direct heat is applied to the body, it causes the vessels in the body to expand, which could increase blood loss and worsen the patient's condition. Choices 1, 3, and 4 are incorrect because when a patient is going into shock, you should prevent more blood loss, administer intravenous fluids, and prevent the loss of body heat.

3. **The correct answer is 1.** Lister scissors, which are angled and have blunt tips, are made for cutting bandages. Choice 2 is incorrect because Carless scissors are used to cut sutures. Choices 3 and 4 are incorrect because Mayo and Metzenbaum scissors are used to cut or dissect soft tissue.

4. **The correct answer is 3.** Chest tubes used for drainage are placed between the ribs, usually at the seventh or eighth intercostal space. Choices 1 and 2 are incorrect because these choices indicate spaces too high on the chest. Choice 4 is incorrect because it indicates a space too low on the chest.

5. **The correct answer is 1.** Fluorescein staining is a preoperative diagnostic test that can help determine whether a patient has damage of the cornea. Choice 2 is incorrect because electroretinography tests whether a patient has damage of the retina. Choice

3 is incorrect because the Schirmer tear test tests tear production. Choice 4 is incorrect because ultrasonography can identify many different conditions, but not damaged corneas.

6. **The correct answer is 2.** Adson forceps are classified as dissecting forceps. Choice 1 is incorrect because Littlewood forceps are tissue forceps. Choice 3 is incorrect because Ruskin forceps are bone cutting forceps. Choice 4 is incorrect because Babcock forceps are intestinal tissue forceps.

7. **The correct answer is 4.** Instruments used during surgery should be cleaned as soon as possible after surgery so that blood, saline, and other liquids do not corrode the instruments. Choice 1 is incorrect because sharp items, such as scalpels, should be removed from the instrument tray first. Choice 2 is incorrect because delicate surgical instruments should be cleaned separately from other surgical instruments. Choice 3 is incorrect because instruments should be scrubbed under warm water without using abrasive brushes.

8. **The correct answer is 1.** If a surgeon asks one of the scrubbed team members to pick up a sterile instrument from the tray, acceptable aseptic techniques are being followed because a sterile team member is handling a sterile instrument. Choice 2 is incorrect because a nonsterile team member should not reach across a sterilized area. Choice 3 is incorrect because all members of the surgical team should face toward each other and the sterilized area. Choice 4 is incorrect because sterile tables should be draped with water-resistant fabric.

9. **The correct answer is 3.** Large adult dogs, such as a golden retriever, should fast for 6–12 hours before surgery. Large dogs can handle a longer fasting time period than small or young dogs because their glycogen reserves are larger. Choices

1 and 2 are incorrect because large dogs should fast for longer time periods. Choice 4 is incorrect because the time period is too long.

10. **The correct answer is 4.** The first step in preparing a patient for surgery is evacuating the bladder. Once the bladder has been evacuated, the veterinary technician may begin clipping hair or fur from the site, choice 3. After clipping, the technician should continue by protecting the site from nearby hair by wrapping the paw or foot, choice 2. Finally, the technician can then begin scrubbing for sterilization, choice 1.

SUMMING IT UP

- Surgical preparation and assisting questions are multiple-choice questions, incomplete statements, and scenarios that require your knowledge of surgical procedures, surgical instruments, sterilization techniques, and operating room procedures.

- You should also be familiar with the anatomies of different animals, medical terminology, patient positioning, suturing techniques, and more.

- When answering surgical preparation and assisting questions, remember that all surgical procedures are different, sterilization is key, and every instrument has a purpose. Also, read each question carefully, paying close attention to the way the questions are worded.

CHAPTER 6

Laboratory Procedures Questions

OVERVIEW

- **Preparing for laboratory procedures questions**
- **Tips for answering laboratory procedures questions**
- **Practice questions**
- **Answer key and explanations**
- **Summing it up**

PREPARING FOR LABORATORY PROCEDURES QUESTIONS

Another group of questions on the VTNE involves laboratory procedures. These questions make up 15 percent (30 items) of the questions on the exam. These questions test your knowledge of collecting specimens or samples, preparing samples for lab tests, performing the lab tests and procedures, and maintaining safety in the lab.

Laboratory procedures questions may ask you to identify the correct definition of a named procedure or to select the correct use of a particular tool or piece of equipment. You might have to identify a correct or incorrect statement among four choices. You may also encounter questions that describe a scenario and ask you how the technician in the description should proceed.

To answer these types of questions, you have to rely on what you know about anatomy, bodily fluids, and common laboratory tests and procedures. You may be asked questions about the process of gathering specimens (e.g., drawing blood, collecting urine or feces, retrieving parasites, etc.) or you may be asked about the results of laboratory tests (e.g., what the sample would look like if it tested positive for the presence of a specific disease).

COMMONLY USED LAB EQUIPMENT/INSTRUMENTS

- Bunsen burners
- Centrifuges
- Compound microscopes
- Crucibles
- Evaporating discs
- Forceps
- Glass and plastic bottles

- Measuring cylinders
- Mortar and pestles
- Needles
- Pipettes
- Rubber stoppers
- Test tubes
- Vacutainers

Some laboratory procedures questions focus on one of the most commonly used pieces of equipment in veterinary laboratories—the microscope. You may be asked about specific parts of a microscope (e.g., where a part is located or what its function is) or how to care for a microscope (e.g., how it is stored, how it is cleaned).

Laboratory procedures questions can be based on a multitude of subjects. Questions in this group generally cover topics including:

Common animal diseases

Medical terms

Toxicology

Preparing, storing, and dispensing biological and chemical agents

Aseptic and sterilization techniques for equipment and supplies

Sample collection, preparation, storing, and shipping techniques

Laboratory diagnostic principles and procedures

Reading laboratory and diagnostic test results

Inventory control

Record keeping

To prepare for these questions, study information related to these topics. Also, remember to review the anatomy of the most common animals that small-animal and large-animal veterinarians treat. Study the most common types of tests performed in veterinary laboratories, including the reasons for why these tests are ordered and how normal and abnormal results are determined. Familiarize yourself with the most commonly used lab equipment and tools, and be sure you know how to properly clean and maintain them. Remember that keeping records of your findings in a laboratory and correctly labeling your samples for storage and shipment are also essential to a safe and professional lab environment.

TIPS FOR ANSWERING LABORATORY PROCEDURES QUESTIONS

You will perform well on laboratory procedures questions if you recall the following tips when studying for and taking the test:

1. **Safety first.** Some of the laboratory procedures questions ask about proper sterilization techniques and aseptic techniques. They may ask you about the proper ways to clean laboratory equipment or how to react to a hazardous chemical spill. Sanitation and first aid are popular topics for test questions because the safety of technicians in a lab is important. If you remember that laboratory safety is crucial, you will find it easier to answer questions concerning chemical spills, biological agent exposure, and laboratory accidents.

For example, you are given a scenario in which a veterinary technician breaks a beaker of toxic chemicals. As the beaker drops to the floor, the chemicals splash onto the technician and hits the area of his skin exposed between his gloves and the sleeve of his lab coat. After the bottle breaks, the technician attempts to pick up the glass pieces and cuts himself. What should the veterinary technician do?

Regardless of the options presented to you, you should know the option you are looking for will include actions that will keep the technician safe and address the technician's injuries. You should know that he should not continue to pick up the pieces of glass, as they are sharp and covered in toxic chemical agents. You should also know that he should not put his own safety aside to clean up the mess. The correct answer option will include a description of the technician properly washing the area of skin exposed to the chemicals and tending to his cut. Only after the technician is out of harm's way should he clean the spill.

LABORATORY SAFETY TECHNIQUES

- Monitor the use of quality control samples
- Train technicians thoroughly
- Allow only authorized personnel in the lab
- Prohibit smoking, eating, and drinking
- Require the use of protective lab coats
- Wear goggles and disposable gloves when necessary
- Clean and disinfect work surfaces after procedures

- Clearly label glass and plastic bottles and containers
- Turn off all Bunsen burners when not in use
- Dispose of waste correctly
- Alert all technicians to chemical or other hazardous spills
- Record all laboratory accidents
- Practice inventory control

---

2. **Know the body's fluids and how to collect them.** While studying for the VTNE, focus on the types of fluids typically tested in veterinary labs. These include blood, urine, saliva, cerebrospinal fluid, synovial fluid, thoracic fluid, and peritoneal fluid. Familiarize yourself with what these fluids do and where they are located within the body. What do these fluids look like? What are their colors and consistencies? Do they have distinct smells? Do they change when exposed to the air? From which area of the body would you obtain these fluids? Does this differ among different species or breeds?

Questions in this group ask you about the steps technicians must perform before, during, and after completing procedures. They may ask you about the best positions in which to place a dog when drawing blood, or they may ask you which size needle you should use to draw a specific fluid. Questions about which laboratory tests you would perform if you were looking for a specific disease or using a certain fluid are also included in this group. You will score higher on the VTNE if you know the most common lab tests and the techniques for obtaining the different bodily fluids.

Another topic you should focus on while preparing for laboratory procedures questions on the VTNE is interpreting the results of lab tests. Some questions on the exam will describe a procedure and ask what the results of that procedure should tell you about the animal. Others will ask you about results that may indicate something went wrong in the testing process.

COMMON LABORATORY TESTS AND PROCEDURES

- Abdominocentesis
- Allergy testing
- Chemistry panel surveys
- Colorimetry
- Complete blood counts
- Fine-needle aspirates
- Fungal culture
- Heartworm test
- Hemoglobin estimation

- Histopathology
- Necropsy
- Parasite exams
- Skin scraping
- Thyroid function tests
- Toxicology
- Urinalysis
- Virology

For example, you are told that a technician has received a test tube filled with plasma obtained from a cat. The color of the plasma is a dark red. The technician knows the plasma should be either transparent or a light pink. The technician suspects in vitro hemolysis. You are then asked to identify a cause of in vitro hemolysis in the answer options.

To answer this question, you have to know that hemolysis is a process in which red blood cells break, releasing their contents into the plasma or serum. Hemolysis can occur inside the body, but is most commonly the result of poor lab work. You should know osmotic pressure, the size of the needle, the failure to separate plasma, and the vigorous mixing of samples can cause red cells to break and spill into the plasma. Look for one of these causes within the answer choices.

3. **Look for specific details.** One of the easiest ways to choose incorrect answers on the VTNE is to misunderstand what the question is asking you. This is especially common in laboratory procedure questions because some questions are about techniques, some are about the animals themselves, and others are about laboratory rules and safety. This group features such a wide variety of questions that it is easy to get confused. If you take your time, read the question thoroughly, and then read each answer choice, you should be able to choose the correct answers.

You should evaluate certain answer choices more closely depending on what the question is asking you to determine. You may need to focus on the equipment used in a particular scenario. Or, you may have to focus on the behavior of the animal. Sometimes, you may even have to assess the reaction of the client or owner. Once you understand what the question is asking you, go back to the beginning and reread the question looking for important details.

Beware of questions that include the word *except*. If you skip over this word in a question, you may be confused by the answer options. This may result in either spending too much time on one question or choosing the incorrect answer. You should also pay attention to the specific species or breed included in the scenario or question. Other important details may include the age or sex of the animal, as these details may change the way a technician performs procedures or interprets results.

PRACTICE QUESTIONS

1. A gray and red Vacutainer tube contains:
   1. heparin.
   2. silicone serum separation material.
   3. thrombin.
   4. silicone coating with no additive.

2. When performing venipuncture on a cat using the left femoral vein, the patient should be placed in:
   1. dorsal recumbency.
   2. right lateral recumbency.
   3. left lateral recumbency.
   4. sternal recumbency.

3. Arthrocentesis is the method used to collect:
   1. abdominal fluid.
   2. cerebrospinal fluid.
   3. synovial fluid.
   4. thoracic fluid.

4. A healthy feline should have a red blood cell count ranging from:
   1. 5.0–$8.5 \times 10^6/mm^3$.
   2. 5.5–$9.5 \times 10^6/mm^3$.
   3. 5.5–$10.0 \times 10^6/mm^3$.
   4. 7.0–$13.0 \times 10^6/mm^3$.

5. A veterinarian collects a blood sample from a ferret to check the animal's WBC count. This sample will provide information about the ferret's:
   1. white blood cells.
   2. whole blood cells.
   3. white blood culture.
   4. whole blood culture.

6. Hemolysis is a form of cell disintegration in:
   1. white blood cells.
   2. red blood cells.
   3. platelets.
   4. plasma.

7. A postprandial urine sample would be taken after a period of:
   1. activity.
   2. rest.
   3. eating.
   4. fasting.

8. Which of the following technicians is violating laboratory safety procedures?
   1. Bill uses small- and medium-sized containers instead of large containers to store chemicals in the laboratory.
   2. Joseph wears a protective coat, disposable gloves, and goggles while working with chemical agents.
   3. Amanda accidentally ingests a biological agent and seeks the aid of the senior lab technician.
   4. Tiffany breaks a beaker of toxic substances, cleans up the spill and the broken glass, and goes back to work.

9. The majority of clinical waste disposal containers are which color?
   1. Purple
   2. Blue
   3. Green
   4. Red

10. All the following are common anticoagulants *except*:
    1. sodium citrate.
    2. heparin.
    3. zeolite.
    4. EDTA.

ANSWER KEY AND EXPLANATIONS

1. 2	3. 3	5. 1	7. 3	9. 4
2. 3	4. 3	6. 2	8. 4	10. 3

1. **The correct answer is 2.** A gray and red Vacutainer tube contains silicone serum separation material. This type of Vacutainer is also known as a Serum Separation Tube. Green Vacutainer tubes contain heparin, choice 1. Yellow and gray Vacutainer tubes contain thrombin, choice 3. Red and yellow Vacutainer tubes contain a silicone coating with no additive, choice 4.

2. **The correct answer is 3.** When performing venipuncture on a cat using the left femoral vein, the patient should be placed in left lateral recumbency. With the patient in this position, the restrainer can occlude the vein by pressing on the medial side of the upper thigh with one hand. None of the positions in choices 1, 2, or 4 would be useful for this procedure, so these options are incorrect.

3. **The correct answer is 3.** Arthrocentesis is the method used to collect synovial fluid from joints to help examine joint problems such as lameness or arthritis. This method is not used to collect abdominal fluid, cerebrospinal fluid, or thoracic fluid, so choices 1, 2, and 4 are incorrect.

4. **The correct answer is 3.** A healthy feline should have a red blood cell count ranging from 5.5–10.0 RBCs. Choice 1 is incorrect because it indicates the red blood cell count of a dog. Choices 2 and 4 are incorrect because these options indicate the red blood cell counts of an equine and a thoroughbred, respectively.

5. **The correct answer is 1.** The blood sample will check the ferret's white blood cells. The abbreviation WBC stands for white blood cells. Choices 2, 3, and 4 are incorrect because the abbreviation WBC does not stand for whole blood cells, white blood culture, or whole blood culture.

6. **The correct answer is 2.** Hemolysis involves the deterioration of red blood cells. During this process, red blood cells break and release their contents into the plasma or serum that has been extracted

from the animal. Hemolysis is typically visible, as the fluids in the test tube are a dark red color rather than a pink color or clear. Choices 1, 3, and 4 are incorrect because hemolysis does not affect the white blood cells, platelets, or technically the plasma. Although the breaking of the red blood cells influences the plasma, the effect of hemolysis is indirect.

7. **The correct answer is 3.** A postprandial urine sample would be taken after a period of eating. This form of urine collection would produce a sample that would be reflective of the patient's diet. A sample taken after a period of activity, choice 1, would have a low level of concentration. A sample taken after a period of rest, choice 2, would be highly concentrated. A sample taken after a period of fasting, choice 4, would be free of any dietary effects.

8. **The correct answer is 4.** Tiffany violated laboratory safety procedures when she went back to work without recording or reporting the incident. When spills occur in labs, no matter the substance spilled or where it took place, the incident should always be recorded. Choice 1 is incorrect because small- and medium-sized containers in labs cut down on the occurrence of large spills. Choice 2 is incorrect because Joseph is fully prepared to deal with all chemical and biological agents. Choice 3 is incorrect because Amanda, unsure of what to do in her situation, turns to a superior for guidance, thus alerting the staff to the situation and seeking medical help.

9. **The correct answer is 4.** The majority of clinical waste disposal containers in the United States are red. Some laboratories and clinics may choose to color code their waste containers and some clinics use yellow containers for radiation waste; however, most clinics' containers are red. Choices 1, 2, and

3 are incorrect since the majority of waste disposal bins are not purple, blue, or green.

10. **The correct answer is 3.** Zeolite is an absorbent chemical used to help seal various bodily injuries and is considered a procoagulant, rather than an anticoagulant. Choices 1, 2, and 4 are incorrect because sodium citrate, heparin, and EDTA are common anticoagulants used in veterinary medicine. Another common anticoagulant is oxalate fluoride.

SUMMING IT UP

- Laboratory procedures questions on the VTNE test your knowledge of collecting specimens and samples, preparing samples for lab tests, performing the lab tests and procedures, and maintaining safety in the lab.

- Be sure to study the most common procedures and processes completed in laboratory settings. Also, be familiar with the most common equipment and instruments used in laboratories, as well as the anatomy of patients most commonly treated by veterinarians.

- Be able to identify safety hazards in laboratory settings. Familiarize yourself with safety rules and regulations, including what to do in case of a spill or injury. Remember that the technician's safety is a main priority and should not be overlooked or ignored.

- Understand all the steps that must be completed before testing specimens. This includes collecting specimens, withdrawing bodily fluids, and stabilizing or positioning the patient. Familiarize yourself with characteristics of the specimens that technicians regularly use to perform tests. Study the different outcomes of each procedure.

- Carefully read each question on the VTNE and look for specific details that may help you answer laboratory procedures questions. The species, breed, age, and sex of an animal may change the way you perform tests or interpret results.

CHAPTER 7

Animal Care and Nursing Questions

OVERVIEW

- **Preparing for animal care and nursing questions**
- **Tips for answering animal care and nursing questions**
- **Practice questions**
- **Answer key and explanations**
- **Summing it up**

PREPARING FOR ANIMAL CARE AND NURSING QUESTIONS

Animal care and nursing is the next domain on the VTNE. This section includes 24 percent (48 items) of the questions on the exam; therefore, this is the most common type of question you'll have to answer when taking the exam. These multiple-choice questions will test your knowledge of performing and documenting evaluations of patients' physical, behavioral, and nutritional statuses. To answer these questions correctly, you'll need to know how to perform many nursing and clinical diagnostic procedures, such as wound management and pre- and postoperative care.

Animal care and nursing questions may ask you to choose the correct definition of a named procedure, to identify the correct vein from which to draw blood from a certain animal, or to select the correct use of a particular piece of equipment. Other questions might ask you to indicate which of four statements is accurate and true.

This domain calls upon your knowledge of a wide variety of topics, from providing comfort and support to recovering patients to sterilizing equipment and performing simple diagnostic procedures. What you know about an animal's body and behavior will help you in this section of the test. To answer these questions, you should also know about setting up animal cages and performing triage. You may be asked questions about the process of preparing an animal for surgery, ways to educate the public about disease control, or the correct ways to keep records.

Some questions in this domain may ask you about caring for patients that arrive at clinics with their owners after accidents. The types of accidents you will see range from inadvertent poisonings to internal damages after being struck by vehicles. When a patient comes in, you'll immediately have to perform triage, or determine treatments based on the severity of the patient's condition. Questions that ask about patient triage will most likely present you with a scenario in which an animal has been injured or is ill and then will ask you to categorize the patient's condition. Categories are typically: none (nonemergency), minor (mild emergency), urgent (serious emergency), critical (life-threatening emergency), and catastrophic (no survival even with treatment).

Some of the animal care and nursing questions on the VTNE also ask you about bandaging techniques. Many of the animals you'll examine in the field or in clinics have wounds that need to be treated. You must know how to properly disinfect, suture, and bandage wounds. When dealing with bandage questions, you'll be asked about materials commonly used in bandages, techniques to bandaging particular animal body parts, and ways to ensure the technician's, nurse's, and client's safety when bandaging an animal.

BANDAGING/DRESSING TECHNIQUES

- Avian bandaging
- Ball bandaging
- Carpal flexion bandages
- Cohesive bandages
- Compression bandages
- Crepe bandages
- Dry dressings
- Figure 8 bandaging
- Haemostatic dressings
- Impregnated gauze dressings
- Interdigitating bandaging
- Occlusive dressings
- Robert Jones bandaging
- Sugar/honey bandaging
- Tie-over dressing
- Tubular bandages
- White open wave bandages

Animal care and nursing questions cover a wide range of topics. Some of these topics include:

Aseptic, sterilization, and disinfectant techniques

Disease control and preventative techniques

Environmental health/safety procedures

Animal husbandry

Animal nutrition

Pre- and postoperative care

Bandaging and wound management

Simple diagnostic procedures

Public health

Forming relationships with patients and with clients

Preparing clinics for animal residency

Inventory control

Record keeping

While preparing for these questions, focus on studying information related to these topics. Also, remember to review the anatomy of the most common animals that small-animal and large-animal veterinarians treat. Study the most common types of wound management techniques and diagnostic procedures, including the reasons why procedures are ordered and treatments are administered. Familiarize yourself with the most commonly used instruments in the clinic and be sure you know how to disinfect them and the surfaces on which they are used. Remember that keeping accurate records of patient visits is also a critical portion of animal care. If a record is inaccurate and is given to someone other than the attending or receiving veterinarian without legal documentation, ethical issues may arise.

TIPS FOR ANSWERING ANIMAL CARE AND NURSING QUESTIONS

You will perform well on animal care and nursing questions if you recall the following tips when studying for and taking the test:

1. **Provide a comfortable environment.** Many questions in this domain of the VTNE will ask you about the environments in which veterinary offices and clinics should house patients. Patients may stay overnight at clinics before or after an operation, and they may need to be closely monitored. If an animal is comfortable in its environment, it will recover faster. When you're presented with questions like these, remember to look for the answer that offers the animal the greatest relief or the most comfort.

Some questions pertaining to the comfort of patients may require you to know about particular species' preferences of bedding and food. For example, cats typically behave better and recover faster if they have some privacy, so nurses or technicians often place cat cages out of the sight of other animals. If their cages cannot be moved, then technicians often place blankets or sheets over the cages to give the animals the privacy they desire.

COMMON PRODUCTS IN VETERINARY CLINICS

- Air filtration units
- Anesthesia machines and masks
- Aquariums
- Catheter kits
- Dog/cat toys
- Handling gloves
- Heartworm test kits
- Hematology analyzer

- Kennels
- Microscopes
- Mobility carts
- Palpation sleeves
- Pet stairs/ramps
- Stainless steel cages
- Restraint collars/muzzles
- Vital signs monitors

Although many of the questions on the VTNE deal with common pets such as dogs, cats, rabbits, birds, and ferrets, you also need to be prepared to answer animal care and nursing questions about farm animals, exotic animals, and reptiles. For example, you may be asked to identify the most appropriate materials a technician or nurse would use to line the cage of an iguana, and you would have to know that alfalfa pellets are the correct material.

Questions concerning the comfort and safety of animals held in a clinic may require you to recall information about temperatures in which specific animals thrive (e.g., cats recover better in facilities kept at a temperature above 50°F). They may also require you to know the reasons why specific procedures are followed.

2. **Ethical dilemmas.** Some animal care and nursing questions on the VTNE are based on the American Veterinary Medical Association (AVMA) Code of Ethics or the Veterinary Technician Code of Ethics. These questions require you to choose the most ethical response to a problem or situation involving public health, veterinarian-client-patient relationships, and veterinarian-client privileges. For these questions, you may be presented with a scenario and asked to respond ethically.

For example, a client who has profited immensely from breeding her prized French mastiff approaches a veterinarian with a favor to ask. She tells the veterinarian that her dog has recently had puppies, but one of them has a clear case of entropion. She asks the veterinarian if he can fix the puppy's eye so she can sell the puppy for the maximum amount. How should the veterinarian respond?

When reading the answer options to this type of question, you should immediately eliminate those that feature the veterinarian behaving unethically. This includes bargaining with the client for a cut of the profits, speaking to the client disrespectfully, and even performing the procedure. According to the AVMA Code of Ethics, it is unethical to perform a surgery to fix a genetic defect or condition, such as entropion, in animals that are going to be shown, sold, bred, or raced. Your knowledge of the AVMA's Code of Ethics will allow you to answer questions concerning ethical dilemmas.

PRINCIPLES OF VETERINARY MEDICAL ETHICS

- Veterinarians should consider the needs of the patient above all else.

- Nurses, technicians, and veterinarians should remain honest, fair, and respectful of the patient and the client.

- Both the veterinarian and the client must agree to start a veterinarian-client-patient relationship. Either party can end the relationship in the future.

- Any veterinarian who doesn't believe that he/she can adequately treat a patient with a specific condition should refer the client to a fellow specialist who can.

- All veterinarians are encouraged to collaborate with other technicians, nurses, and specialists to develop the best care for their patients.

- All associates working in a veterinary clinic or hospital should protect the rights of their patients and clients at all times.

To read the AVMA's Principles of Veterinary Medical Ethics, visit www.avma.org.

Other ethical dilemmas you'll most likely encounter on the VTNE include appropriate record keeping, dispersal of privileged information, irresponsible inventory control, and poor or inappropriate communication among veterinarians and their coworkers or clients. Studying the AVMA Code of Ethics and the Veterinary Technician's Code of Ethics will help you answer professional ethics questions in this domain.

3. Keep a positive attitude. A technician's or nurse's attitude affects the level of care provided to animals at clinics and hospitals; therefore, questions about the appropriate attitude and behavior of nurses, technicians, and veterinarians are common in this domain.

As you may recall, a nurse's mood can affect the mood of many of the animals in his or her care. For example, rabbits often become tense when the nurse caring for them is stressed or upset. Evaluating and treating a tense rabbit is more difficult, and more dangerous, than treating a calm one. This applies to pets such as cats and dogs too. When speaking to animals in a clinic, especially those in recovery, caregivers should always use a low, gentle voice. Technicians should also frequently pet and groom the animals. This attention makes animals feel comforted and special and may aid in their recovery. High, shrill noises and rough touches will cause the patient to feel upset or stressed, which may prolong its recovery or cause further injury or illness.

To answer these questions, remember to use common sense and look for options that feature nurses or technicians treating patients respectfully. While the caregiver should be gentle, there may be times in which they must be firm. When this is the case, the answer option shouldn't include physical abuse to the animal or sharp, angry words.

Keeping a positive attitude and speaking gently, yet firmly, to patients affects the patients' care, but it also keeps the caregiver safe. When animals are excited, angry, or tense, they may attack the caregiver. This is especially true when technicians or nurses attempt to restrain injured animals. The best way to restrain an animal is to crouch down to the patient's eye level, speak to it gently, and call it forward. Be sure to avoid eye contact, as many animals see this as threatening behavior. Also avoid sitting in front of the animal because if the animal chooses to attack, this position leaves you vulnerable.

PRACTICE QUESTIONS

1. A canine patient presents with excessively greasy skin, diffuse scaling, erythema, alopecia, and inflammation. Which of the following is the most likely diagnosis?
   1. Fleas
   2. Ringworm
   3. Demodectic mange
   4. Seborrhea oleosa

2. A dog that was hit by a car and is now recovering from surgery appears to have lost its appetite. When the caregiver sets the food in front of the dog, it does not show an interest in the food. Which of the following is true of animals that have been injured or have diseases?
   1. Their metabolic rate increases, and they become severely nutritionally compromised after a few days without food.
   2. Their metabolic rate decreases, and they become severely nutritionally compromised after only one day without food.
   3. Their metabolic rate increases, and they become severely nutritionally compromised after only one day without food.
   4. Their metabolic rate decreases, and they become severely nutritionally compromised after a few days without food.

3. A zoonotic disease is one that:
   1. is not contagious or life threatening.
   2. only affects those animals kept in zoos.
   3. is only common in undeveloped countries.
   4. can be transmitted from animals to humans.

4. Bandaged animals often bite at the bandages if they are uncomfortable (too loose or too tight) or if the animal is simply bored. Many times, these bandages are pressure bandages applied by surgeons after an operation. Pressure bandages should be removed how many hours after application?
   1. 4 hours
   2. 8 hours
   3. 12 hours
   4. 18 hours

5. Which of the following steps would a veterinary technician perform *last* when inserting an intravenous catheter?
   1. Palpate the animal's lymph nodes
   2. Administer drugs slowly and carefully
   3. Examine the catheter site for infections
   4. Wash hands with antibacterial/disinfectant soaps

6. Which of the following ECG findings is a sign of third-degree AV block?
   1. No P waves and wide distorted QRS complexes
   2. Lengthening of PR interval on consecutive beats
   3. Constant PR interval with random dropped beats
   4. No relation between P waves and QRS complexes

7. Horner's Syndrome is a temporary condition that *most* commonly affects a cat's:
   1. facial nerves.
   2. esophagus.
   3. adrenal gland.
   4. spinal cord.

8. A veterinarian suspects that a herd of cattle is suffering from molybdenum poisoning because their milk production has decreased, the color of their coats is fading, and they appear to be losing weight. This condition should be categorized as:
   1. a nonemergency.
   2. minor.
   3. serious.
   4. life threatening.

9. A client seeks the professional services of a new veterinarian for her pet without a referral. The new veterinarian calls the former veterinarian to discuss the patient's medical history. The former veterinarian should:
   1. share information with the new veterinarian.
   2. report the new veterinarian for stealing a patient from him.
   3. withhold information from the new veterinarian because it is privileged.
   4. keep information from the new veterinarian because he did not make a referral.

10. Humane euthanasia of animals is:
    1. rare.
    2. illegal.
    3. ethical.
    4. unethical.

ANSWER KEY AND EXPLANATIONS

1. 4	3. 4	5. 2	7. 1	9. 1
2. 1	4. 3	6. 4	8. 3	10. 3

1. **The correct answer is 4.** Seborrhea oleosa presents with excessively greasy skin, diffuse scaling, erythema, alopecia, and inflammation. Infestation with fleas (choice 1) would result in itching, crusty skin, alopecia, and flea dirt. Ringworm (choice 2) would present with alopecia in circular patches, sometimes with dry, crusty skin. Demodectic mange (choice 3) would present with areas of red and scaly lesions around the face and front legs.

2. **The correct answer is 1.** Injured or diseased animals may experience an increased metabolic rate and their bodies may become severely nutritionally compromised after a few days without food. These patients may need to be assisted orally during feedings or they may receive a gastrosomy tube. Their water intake should also be monitored. Choices 2 and 4 are incorrect because these options state that the metabolic rate decreases, which is untrue. Choice 3 is incorrect because the patient's body becomes nutritionally compromised after a few days without food, not over the course of one day.

3. **The correct answer is 4.** A zoonotic disease is contagious and may be transmitted from animals to humans or from humans to animals (this is called reverse zoonosis). Examples of zoonotic diseases include Ebola virus, cowpox, rabies, and the bird flu. Many scientists suspect SARS may be a form of a zoonotic disease as well. Choice 1 is incorrect because zoonotic diseases are contagious and may be life threatening, depending on the patient and the type of virus. Choice 2 is incorrect because these viruses can and do infect animals outside of zoos. Choice 3 is incorrect because these diseases also affect animals and humans living in developed countries.

4. **The correct answer is 3.** Pressure bandages should be removed approximately 12 hours after they are applied. After 12 hours, pressure bandages may become uncomfortable, which may lead the animal to bite at the material. If the material breaks, bacteria from the animal's mouth and exposure to environmental elements may infect the wound. Choices 1 and 2 are incorrect because the bandage typically will not irritate the animal within this time period. Choice 4 is incorrect because pressure bandages should not remain on animals past 12 hours.

5. **The correct answer is 2.** Veterinary technicians should administer drugs slowly and carefully into the animal only after they have washed their hands with disinfectant soaps (choice 4), examined the catheter site for infections (choice 3), and palpated the animal's lymph nodes (choice 1). Choices 1, 3, and 4 are incorrect because these steps should be completed before moving on to administering the drugs.

6. **The correct answer is 4.** An ECG of a patient with third-degree heart block will demonstrate no relation between P waves and QRS complexes. In this condition, the atria and the ventricles are beating independently of one another. An ECG that shows no P waves and wide distorted QRS complexes (choice 1) indicates premature ventricular contractions. An ECG that shows a lengthening of PR interval on consecutive beats (choice 2) indicates second-degree heart block. An ECG showing a constant PR interval with random dropped beats (choice 3) would also indicate second-degree heart block.

7. **The correct answer is 1.** Horner's Syndrome is caused by a variety of circumstances such as injury to nerves during the surgery, bites to the face, or accidents injuring the head or neck. It affects a cat's facial nerves and causes drooping and a sunken appearance of the eye on one side of the face. It usually resolves itself in 6–8 weeks. Choices 2, 3, and 4 are incorrect because these are not affected by Horner's Syndrome.

8. **The correct answer is 3.** Although molybdenum poisoning is not a life-threatening condition, it is still a serious emergency. This condition is not

life threatening because it can be easily treated. Molybdenum is typically found in clovers; therefore, farmers should direct the herd to graze in areas without clover. Choices 1, 2, and 4 are incorrect because this condition is a serious emergency. An example of a nonemergency would be an insect bite, an example of a minor emergency would be vomiting, and a life-threatening emergency would be internal bleeding or similar injuries.

9. **The correct answer is 1.** Although the client did not ask for a referral and did not formally end the veterinarian-client-patient relationship, the former veterinarian should still share information about the patient with the new veterinarian. According to the AVMA Code of Ethics, the veterinarian should treat the situation as though there had been a referral. Choice 2 is incorrect because there is no proof that the new veterinarian forced the patient to switch, nor did the patient end the previous relationship with the old veterinarian. Choice 3 is incorrect because the information is not privileged in this situation. Choice 4 is incorrect because a referral is not necessary.

10. **The correct answer is 3.** Humane euthanasia of animals is ethical. When an animal is too ill or has sustained injuries from which they cannot possibly recover, veterinarians may recommend that the client consent to euthanizing his or her pet. According to the AVMA Code of Ethics, when humane techniques are used, this process is ethical. Choices 1, 2, and 3 are incorrect because euthanasia is not rare, illegal, or unethical.

SUMMING IT UP

- Animal care and nursing questions test your knowledge of performing and documenting initial and ongoing evaluations of the patient's physical, behavioral, and nutritional status to provide for optimal safety and health.

- Review everything you know about the anatomy of patients most commonly treated by veterinarians. Understand common areas for injections and specimen withdrawal.

- Understand the different categories of animal emergencies and be able to recognize examples of each. Be prepared to answer questions about the most common animal injuries, illnesses, and diseases.

- Know the elements that make a clinical environment comfortable for an animal that may be recovering from an injury, illness, or procedure. Be sure to review facts about animal behaviors and eating habits. Understand disinfecting, sterilization, and aseptic processes and how to maintain a clean, sterile environment.

- Thoroughly review the AVMA Code of Ethics and the Veterinary Technician's Code of Ethics. Familiarize yourself with the aspects of a successful veterinarian-client-patient relationship.

- Recall that positive attitudes and calm environments help patients heal quicker. Sudden, loud noises should be kept to a minimum in veterinary clinics, and nurses and technicians should always speak to their patients in low, calm voices. Nurses and technicians should feed and groom patients frequently and remove any urine or feces from their cages or kennels as soon as possible.

CHAPTER 8

Anesthesia and Analgesia Questions

OVERVIEW

- Preparing for anesthesia and analgesia questions
- Tips for answering anesthesia and analgesia questions
- Practice questions
- Answers and explanations
- Summing it up

PREPARING FOR ANESTHESIA AND ANALGESIA QUESTIONS

Anesthesia and analgesia questions make up another group of questions on the VTNE. This group accounts for 15 percent (30 items) of the questions on the exam. These questions test your knowledge of general, regional, and local anesthesia. Questions on the test will ask how the medications work, when and how they are administered, and how to recognize the different stages and planes of anesthesia.

Anesthesia and analgesia questions may also ask you about the preanesthetic screening process; anesthesia machines and equipment; monitoring techniques prior to, during, and after administering anesthesia; and pain management. They may ask you the differences between administering anesthesia to small animals and administering it to large animals, so you should be familiar with the anatomies of different types of animals such as cats, dogs, horses, cattle, pigs, goats, lizards, snakes, rabbits, birds, ferrets, and guinea pigs.

Anesthesia and analgesia questions may ask you to identify the depth, stage, or plane of anesthesia on a patient based on a definition, statement, or scenario. You may also need to know how certain drugs are administered and why they are administered. The multiple-choice items are formatted as questions, incomplete statements, and scenarios.

You need to know which drugs to administer before, during, and after anesthesia. You also must have knowledge about surgical preparation diagnostic tests that require the use of anesthesia to immobilize animals.

Some questions focus on the rebreathing and non-rebreathing anesthesia machines. You may be asked about the different parts of these machines, the ways they work, the types of animals they are used on, the proper ways to use and maintain them, and the correct procedures to sterilize them.

Anesthesia and analgesia questions are based on many different topics including:

Administering anesthesia	Medical terms
Administering drugs and analgesic medications	Monitoring the animal during anesthesia
Anatomy	Pain assessment
Animal handling	Patient positioning
Aseptic and sterilization techniques for equipment and supplies	Pre- and postanesthetic care
	Pre- and postanesthetic medications
Common animal diseases	Stages of anesthesia
Maintaining and using anesthetic equipment	

To prepare for anesthesia and analgesia questions, remember to study information related to these topics. Remember, veterinarians treat animals of all shapes and sizes, so be sure to familiarize yourself with the different types of animals. Make sure you know how to identify the different depths, stages, and planes of anesthesia and the commonly used anesthetics, sedatives, and analgesics. Review the different anesthetic machines and equipment—including information about their parts and the ways they work.

TIPS FOR ANSWERING ANESTHESIA AND ANALGESIA QUESTIONS

Remember the following tips when answering anesthesia and analgesia questions:

1. **Different animals require different types of anesthesia.** Animals are different and have different anatomies, so the methods of administering anesthesia are not the same for all animals. The animal's age, size, and health must be taken into account before administering anesthesia. For example, due to their complex anatomy, horses must stand during certain procedures and are usually given a local anesthesia combined with heavy sedation. These types of questions may also ask what anesthesia methods and medications are required for different types of animals.

2. **Combinations of anesthetics are used.** Many times general anesthetics are combined with local anesthetics, sedatives, and analgesics. Remember, anesthesia can be inhaled or given intravenously. Local anesthetics and analgesics are used to control pain, while sedatives are used to relax the patient. These types of questions may ask you the names of medications used in conjunction with anesthesia, or they may ask you what conditions specific medications are used to treat. Either way, make sure you know the difference between anesthetics, sedatives, and analgesics.

COMMONLY USED ANESTHETICS, SEDATIVES, AND ANALGESICS

• Acepromazine	• Diazepam	• Medetomidine
• Acetaminophen	• Etomidate	• Midazolam
• Barbiturates	• Halothane	• Opiates
• Bupivicaine	• Isoflurane	• Propofol
• Carprofen	• Ketamine	• Tiletamine
• Chlorpromazine	• Ketoprofen	• Xylazine
• Droperidol	• Lidocaine	• Zolazepam

---

f www.facebook.com/careerresource

PRACTICE QUESTIONS

1. Which of the following medications is an opiate?
   1. Fentanyl
   2. Acetaminophen
   3. Ketoprofen
   4. Lidocaine

2. Which of the following procedures would require a local anesthetic?
   1. Removing a tumor
   2. Cleaning a puncture wound
   3. Amputating a limb
   4. Repairing a fractured bone

3. Which of the following medications is given in conjunction with anesthetics to control pain?
   1. Ketorlac
   2. Procaine
   3. Methohexital
   4. Xylamine

4. Epidural anesthesia is used during surgeries involving the:
   1. head.
   2. upper chest.
   3. shoulders.
   4. hind legs.

5. Which of the following laryngoscope blades is primarily used to intubate large animals?
   1. Phillips
   2. Rowson
   3. Miller
   4. Macintosh

6. After anesthesia is administered to a goat, the animal should be positioned with its head:
   1. facing left.
   2. turned up.
   3. facing down.
   4. turned right.

7. Pigs should be deprived of water for how many hours before surgery requiring anesthesia?
   1. 2
   2. 6
   3. 12
   4. 24

8. The non-rebreathing anesthesia machine is used on which of the following animals?
   1. Cattle
   2. Horses
   3. Ferrets
   4. Goats

9. When animals undergo anesthesia, their ventilation is closely monitored. All these factors are assessed during ventilation monitoring *except*:
   1. rate.
   2. tidal volume.
   3. rhythm.
   4. heart beat.

10. A patient's plasma protein level can alter the absorption rate of which of the following anesthetic agents?
    1. Fentanyl
    2. Propofol
    3. Ketamine HCl
    4. Phenobarbital

ANSWERS AND EXPLANATIONS

1. 1	3. 1	5. 2	7. 1	9. 4
2. 2	4. 4	6. 2	8. 3	10. 4

1. **The correct answer is 1.** Fentanyl is an opiate, which is a type of analgesic that affects the central nervous system. Choice 2 is incorrect because acetaminophen is a pain reliever. Choice 3 is incorrect because ketoprofen is a nonsteroidal anti-inflammatory drug (NSAID). Lidocaine is a local anesthetic, so choice 4 is incorrect.

2. **The correct answer is 2.** Cleaning a puncture wound would require a local anesthetic because it's not a major procedure and would not require the patient to be sedated. Choices 1, 3, and 4 are major procedures that would require the patient to be immobile, so these choices are incorrect.

3. **The correct answer is 1.** Ketorolac is a pain reliever given in conjunction with anesthetics. Choices 2, 3, and 4 are incorrect because procaine is an anesthetic, methohexital is a barbiturate, and xylamine is an emetic drug used to induce vomiting.

4. **The correct answer is 4.** Epidural anesthesia is a type of regional anesthesia that is produced by the injection of a local anesthetic into the epidural space of the lumbar or sacral region of the spine. Choices 1, 2, and 3 are incorrect because epidural anesthesia is not used for surgeries involving the head, upper chest, or shoulders.

5. **The correct answer is 2.** The Rowson laryngoscope blade is used primarily to intubate large animals such as cattle, sheep, and pigs. Choices 1, 3, and 4 are incorrect because Phillips, Miller, and Macintosh blades are not used to intubate large animals.

6. **The correct answer is 2.** After receiving anesthesia, a goat should be held with its head facing up to prevent regurgitation until the endotracheal tube is placed. The goat's head should not be turned left, down, or right because this can cause the goat to regurgitate and block its airway, so choices 1, 3, and 4 are incorrect.

7. **The correct answer is 1.** A pig should not ingest water for 2 hours before undergoing surgery requiring anesthesia, but a pig should fast for 6 to 8 hours before surgery. Choices 2, 3, and 4 are incorrect because the times indicated are too long.

8. **The correct answer is 3.** A non-rebreathing anesthesia machine is generally used on animals weighing less than 10 pounds, so it would be used on ferrets. A rebreathing anesthesia machine is generally used on animals weighing more than 10 pounds, so it would be used on cattle, horses, and goats. Therefore, choices 1, 2, and 4 are incorrect.

9. **The correct answer is 4.** When monitoring ventilation on a patient, a technician is monitoring the patient's breathing. Although the patient's beat will be monitored, it is not a part of ventilation. The rate, volume, and rhythm of the patient's breaths will be assessed during ventilation monitoring, so choices 1, 2, and 3 are incorrect.

10. **The correct answer is 4.** A patient's plasma protein level can alter the absorption rate of phenobarbital, a barbiturate. This is a common occurrence among barbiturates because of their ability to bind to proteins. Fentanyl, propofol, and ketamine HCI are not affected by plasma protein levels, so choices 1, 2, and 3 are incorrect.

SUMMING IT UP

- Anesthesia and analgesia questions are multiple-choice questions that require you to know the different types of anesthesia, the preanesthetic screening process, and anesthesia machines and equipment.

- You should also be familiar with handling animals, monitoring the animal during anesthesia, assessing an animal's pain during and after a procedure, and the stages of anesthesia.

- When answering anesthesia and analgesia questions, remember that not all animals are the same. Certain animals require different types of anesthesia and methods of receiving anesthesia due to their size, age, or anatomy. Also, it is important for you to know the differences among local anesthetics, sedatives, and analgesics.

Dentistry Questions

OVERVIEW

- **Preparing for dentistry questions**
- **Tips for answering dentistry questions**
- **Practice questions**
- **Answer key and explanations**
- **Summing it up**

PREPARING FOR DENTISTRY QUESTIONS

Dentistry questions are another type of question on the VTNE. This group of questions makes up 8 percent (16 items) of the exam. These questions are designed to test your ability to prepare and maintain the various instruments, equipment, and supplies used in veterinary dentistry. To answer the questions, you also have to know how to assist with a variety of basic dental procedures, how to maintain patients' dental health, and how to assist in the treatment of dental conditions and diseases. These questions also test your ability to educate your clients about their pets' dental health, including about preventative care and post-treatment care.

Dental questions may ask you to correctly identify a piece of equipment or a dental condition based on a given definition or scenario. You may also find questions that ask you to select the correct statement from a series of incorrect statements, or choose the incorrect statement from a series of correct statements. The multiple-choice items are generally formatted as questions, incomplete statements, or scenarios.

Veterinary technicians aid in veterinary dentistry by preparing and maintaining the environment, tools, and supplies used in dental procedures. When you are preparing for dental questions, be sure to study the various types of instruments used in the dental office. You should be able to identify each instrument and list its uses. Be sure that you are familiar with instruments such as manual and mechanical scalers, curettes, periodontal probes, shepherd's hooks, dental and periosteal elevators, and other dental tools. You should also understand the proper methods for sterilizing these tools and the office itself.

Questions that deal with dental procedures will require an understanding of dental anatomy and common dental conditions. You should carefully study basic oral anatomy and tooth anatomy. Try to develop a firm understanding of the parts of the tooth, the various kinds of teeth, their specific functions, tooth-numbering systems, and other anatomical information.

TYPES OF TEETH

- *Incisors:* Used for cutting and nibbling
- *Canines:* Used for holding and tearing
- *Premolars:* Used for cutting, shearing, and holding
- *Molars:* Used for grinding
- *Carnassials:* Used for cutting; larger than premolars

Of course, you will also need to know how various basic procedures, like cleaning, dental radiography, or therapeutic procedures are performed. For these questions, you should familiarize yourself with basic oral hygiene methods, the proper procedures for dental cleaning, techniques for dental radiography, treatments for various basic dental conditions or diseases, and general safety protocols. You should also be familiar with common dental problems like malocclusions, oral lesions, caries, abscessed teeth, gingivitis, periodontitis, resorptive lesions, and others.

Common Dental Problems

- Abscessed teeth
- Caries (cavities)
- Enamel hypoplasia
- Fusion
- Gemini
- Gingival hyperplasia
- Gingivitis
- Impaction
- Lymphocytic/plasmacytic stomatitis
- Malocclusions
- Misdirected teeth
- Oral tumors
- Oronasal fistulas
- Periodontitis
- Resorptive lesions
- Retained deciduous teeth
- Stomatitis
- Tetracycline staining
- Trauma
- Worn teeth

Finally, you will also have to demonstrate your ability to educate clients about their pet's dental health, including preventative care and post-treatment care. Again, you will need to have a solid understanding of basic dental procedures and the general principles of veterinary dental health. You will also need to be familiar with the suggested methods and protocols for home dental care, including tips for brushing, dietary information, the use of chew toys, and more. You may also want to review the basic principles of proper client communication.

Dental questions on the VTNE are based on many different topics including:

Anatomy
Pathophysiology
Common animal diseases
Sterilization techniques and quality assurance for equipment and supplies

Patient positioning techniques
Dentistry procedures
Dental equipment, instruments, and supplies

TIPS FOR ANSWERING DENTISTRY QUESTIONS

Remember the following tips when answering dentistry questions:

1. **Different animals have different needs.** Although most dental questions on the VTNE will likely focus on cats and dogs, you may encounter some questions that involve other species. Remember that different species have different dental anatomy and specific needs. As you answer questions on the VTNE, pay close attention to the species and breeds of animals in the scenarios and questions. These details could change which answers are correct.

2. **Remember what you have learned.** The basic information you have learned in preparing for other types of questions on the VTNE may be helpful for answering dental questions. This is especially true for questions that deal with dental radiography. Veterinary radiography is a significant part of the VTNE in the diagnostic imaging domain and the information you learn while studying for that domain can be very helpful when you encounter a dental radiography question. Use what you have already learned to help you make the right choices.

PRACTICE QUESTIONS

1. While conducting a dental exam on a canine patient, you discover an infection between the gum and one of the patient's molars. Which of the following would be the most likely diagnosis?
   1. Stomatitis
   2. Abscess
   3. Caries
   4. Epulis

2. Which dental instrument measures the depth of the gingival sulcus?
   1. Shepherd's hook
   2. Sickle scaler
   3. Periodontal probe
   4. Curette

3. While examining a canine patient, you find that one half of its jaw is noticeably larger than the other half. This condition is known as:
   1. Oligodonta.
   2. Rostro caudal mandibular.
   3. Anodontia.
   4. Level bite.

4. A ruby sharpening stone should be used with:
   1. either dry or water lubricant.
   2. only water lubricant.
   3. only dry lubricant.
   4. neither dry nor wet lubricant.

5. What size of intraoral film is commonly used for radiography of canines or incisors in dogs?
   1. Size 0 (zero)
   2. Size 2
   3. Size 3
   4. Size 4

6. When applying fluoride, for how long should you leave the substance on the patient's teeth?
   1. 1–4 minutes
   2. 5–9 minutes
   3. 10–14 minutes
   4. 15–18 minutes

7. You are examining a feline patient, and you discover some inflammation of the soft tissue of the oral cavity. This condition is known as:
   1. gingival hyperplasia.
   2. gemini.
   3. stomatitis.
   4. enamel hyperplasia.

8. Which of the following refers to the surface of the tooth facing the animal's nose?
   1. Mesial
   2. Buccal
   3. Occlusal
   4. Rostral

9. Mandibular mesioclusion is considered normal for which canine breed?
   1. German shepherd
   2. Cocker spaniel
   3. Pug
   4. Dalmatian

10. Which of the following dental instruments is used for root planing?
    1. Curette
    2. Sickle scaler
    3. Shepherd's hook
    4. Periodontal probe

ANSWER KEY AND EXPLANATIONS

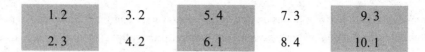

1. 2	3. 2	5. 4	7. 3	9. 3
2. 3	4. 2	6. 1	8. 4	10. 1

1. **The correct answer is 2.** An abscess is described as an infection between the gum and the tooth. Abscesses may also occur at the root of a tooth. Stomatitis (choice 1) presents as an inflammation of the soft tissue in the oral cavity. Caries (choice 3) is another term for a cavity, or tooth decay. Epulis (choice 4) is a nonmalignant oral tumor.

2. **The correct answer is 3.** A periodontal probe measures the depth of the gingival sulcus. A shepherd's hook (choice 1) detects subgingival calculus, cavities, tooth mobility, and broken teeth. A sickle scaler (choice 2) removes supragingival calculus and calculus from other locations. A curette (choice 4) removes subgingival calculus and root planing.

3. **The correct answer is 2.** Rostro caudal mandibular refers to a condition in which the size of one part of the jaw is out of proportion with the other. Oligodonta (choice 1) refers to having fewer teeth than normal. Anodontia (choice 3) refers to having missing teeth. Level bite (choice 4) refers to an end-to-end bite of the incisors.

4. **The correct answer is 2.** A ruby sharpening stone should be used with water lubricant. Choices 1 and 4 are incorrect because a wet lubricant should be used. Choice 3 is incorrect because a dry lubricant should not be used.

5. **The correct answer is 4.** Size 4 intraoral film is used for radiography of canines or incisors in dogs. Size 0 (zero) intraoral film (choice 1) is most commonly used in cats. Size 2 intraoral film (choice 2) is used for many dental X-rays in both cats and dogs. Size 3 intraoral film (choice 3) is not commonly used in veterinary dental radiography.

6. **The correct answer is 1.** Fluoride should be applied to the teeth for about 1–4 minutes. Choices 1, 2, are 4 are incorrect because the times indicated in these choices are too long.

7. **The correct answer is 3.** Inflammation of the soft tissue of the oral cavity is known as stomatitis. Gingival hyperplasia (choice 1) refers to a thickened gingival that occurs as a result of chronic inflammation. Gemini (choice 2) refers to a root that has two crowns. Enamel hyperplasia (choice 4) refers to reduced or missing portions of the enamel.

8. **The correct answer is 4.** Rostral refers to the surface of the tooth facing the animal's nose. Mesial (choice 1) refers to the tooth surface facing the front of the mouth. Buccal (choice 2) refers to the tooth surface facing the cheek. Occlusal (choice 3) refers to the chewing surface of the tooth.

9. **The correct answer is 3.** Mandibular mesioclusion is considered normal for a pug. Pugs are an example of a brachycephalic breed. Brachycephalic dogs have an unusually wide skull and a short maxilla. Mandibular mesioclusion would be considered abnormal in German shepherds, cocker spaniels, and dalmatians (choices 1, 2, and 4) because these breeds are not brachycephalic.

10. **The correct answer is 1.** A curette is used for root planing. A sickle scaler (choice 2) is used for removing calculus. A shepherd's hook (choice 3) is used for detecting calculus, tooth mobility, cavities, broken teeth, and more. A periodontal probe (choice 4) is used to measure the depth of the gingival sulcus.

SUMMING IT UP

- Veterinary technicians often perform duties associated with veterinary dentistry. These duties may include sterilizing and maintaining dental equipment, assisting with dental procedures, performing dental radiography, and educating clients about their pets' dental health.

- Dental questions on the VTNE may cover such topics as dental anatomy, dental instruments, dental procedures, oral hygiene, dental radiography, sterilization and maintenance of dental equipment, dental conditions and treatments, home care, and client education.

- When taking the VTNE, remember that different animal species may have different dental anatomy and dental needs. Also remember that information you have learned for other domains, particularly the diagnostic imaging domain, may be helpful when answering dental questions.

CHAPTER 10

Diagnostic Imaging Questions

OVERVIEW

- Preparing for diagnostic imaging questions
- Tips for answering diagnostic imaging questions
- Practice questions
- Answer key and explanations
- Summing it up

PREPARING FOR DIAGNOSTIC IMAGING QUESTIONS

Diagnostic imaging questions are another type of question on the VTNE. This group of questions makes up about 8 percent (16 items) of the exam. The diagnostic imaging questions on the VTNE are designed to test your knowledge of the various forms of diagnostic imaging, the methods and techniques for using diagnostic imaging devices, X-ray technology, X-ray processing and development techniques, quality assurance techniques, maintenance and safety protocols, positioning techniques, and more.

Diagnostic imaging questions may ask you to correctly identify a piece of equipment or an imaging technique based on a given definition or scenario. You may also find questions that ask you to select the correct statement from a series of incorrect statements or to choose the incorrect statement from a series of correct statements. The multiple-choice items are generally formatted as questions, incomplete statements, or scenarios.

In some cases, a simple physical examination may not be enough for a veterinarian to accurately determine what is wrong with a sick or injured patient. When they need to get a closer look at what is going on inside their patients, technicians frequently use diagnostic imaging tools such as X-rays, MRIs, and ultrasounds to help them in formulating proper diagnoses.

Often, veterinary technicians are responsible for operating the machines that make these images possible. As a potential veterinary technician, you must know how to use diagnostic imaging devices properly so that you can produce high-quality images for the veterinarian.

COMMON DIAGNOSTIC IMAGING TECHNIQUES

- X-ray
- Magnetic resonance imaging (MRI)
- Ultrasound

- Computed tomography (CT) scan
- Nuclear scintigraphy
- Positron emission tomography (PET)

Many of the diagnostic imaging questions on the VTNE will focus on X-ray technology. You will need to familiarize yourself with the science behind X-rays, the components of X-ray machines as well as the machines' functions, the materials used in producing X-rays, processing techniques, the development process, radiographic quality and quality assurance, X-ray safety protocols, patient positioning techniques, and radiographic contrast media.

THE X-RAY DEVELOPMENT PROCESS

- *Developer:* Reduces or converts exposed halide crystals of the X-ray film to black metallic silver

- *Rinse bath:* Stops the development process and prevents contamination of the fixer

- *Fixer:* Removes the unexposed, undeveloped silver halide crystals and hardens the film

- *Wash bath:* Removes processing chemicals and prevents discoloration and fading

- *Drying:* Dries the processed film

To answer diagnostic imaging questions, you'll also need to be familiar with the various forms of digital radiography, such as magnetic resonance imaging (MRI), ultrasound, computed tomography (CT) scans, and more. You will need to know the ways these devices are operated, their diagnostic uses, the types of images they produce, how to interpret these images, and more.

To prepare for questions about ultrasound, you should familiarize yourself with the physics of ultrasound, the ultrasound machine itself, image physics, the ultrasound display, ultrasound artifacts, the sonographic appearance of organs and lesions, and more.

Diagnostic imaging questions on the VTNE are based on many different topics including:

Anatomy
Animal handling and restraining techniques
Diagnostic imaging equipment and procedures
Quality assurance for diagnostic imaging

Environmental health and safety procedures
Procedures for care, maintenance, and use of diagnostic, therapeutic, surgical, and anesthetic equipment and supplies

TIPS FOR ANSWERING DIAGNOSTIC IMAGING QUESTIONS

1. **Know your surroundings.** Diagnostic imaging devices are complex machines that require many different supplies and tools. Be sure you know everything you will need for a typical diagnostic imaging procedure. Be familiar with the various tools and supplies you will be using, remember their functions, and know how to use them properly in all different situations.

2. **Safety first.** As with any medical procedure, safety is your number one concern. Pay close attention to the safety concerns associated with diagnostic imaging procedures, and be sure that both the patient and you remain safe at all times. Ensuring the safety of the patient and other personnel is particularly important when working with X-ray machines. The radiation emitted by X-ray machines can be very dangerous, so it is critically important to be aware of the proper safety protocols for X-ray imaging and ensure that they are observed at all times.

PRACTICE QUESTIONS

1. After soaking in the developer, the next step in developing a radiograph is the:
   1. wash bath.
   2. fixer.
   3. rinse bath.
   4. dryer.

2. Which physical factor may result in diminished radiographic contrast?
   1. Underfiltration
   2. Increased object-film distance
   3. Patient not parallel to the film
   4. Patient too thick

3. A higher grid ratio indicates that:
   1. shorter exposure time is required.
   2. less primary radiation is absorbed.
   3. more scatter radiation is absorbed.
   4. less scatter radiation is absorbed.

4. Which of the following would appear the whitest on an X-ray?
   1. Bone
   2. Organs
   3. Barium
   4. Fat

5. Which of the following problems would result in black marks on a developed radiograph?
   1. Damaged grid
   2. Inadequate rinsing
   3. Debris in cassette
   4. Low processing solutions

6. Which diagnostic imaging technique forms images based on the release of positrons caused by the administration of a radioactive tracer isotope?
   1. CT scan
   2. MRI
   3. Ultrasound
   4. PET scan

7. Which type of ultrasound artifact occurs when sound is completely reflected or absorbed by an object?
   1. Refraction
   2. Acoustic shadowing
   3. Reverberation
   4. Mirror image

8. Dorsoventral is a directional term that indicates an X-ray that enters from the:
   1. back and exits through the abdomen.
   2. tail and exits through the head.
   3. dorsal aspect of the forelimb and exits at the palmar aspect.
   4. dorsal aspect of the hind limb and exits at the plantar aspect.

9. Which of the following processing factors may lead to increased film density?
   1. Improperly mixed developer solution
   2. Incorrect developer temperature
   3. Contaminated developer solution
   4. Diluted developer solution

10. Which of the following is described as a loss of detail due to phosphor variations in the intensifying screen?
    1. Radiographic mottle
    2. Penumbra
    3. Quantum mottle
    4. Structure mottle

ANSWER KEY AND EXPLANATIONS

1. 3	3. 3	5. 1	7. 2	9. 2
2. 1	4. 3	6. 4	8. 1	10. 4

1. **The correct answer is 3.** After the radiograph has been soaked in the developer, it is placed in the rinse bath, which stops the development process and prevents the fixer from becoming contaminated. The wash bath (choice 1) is used after the fixer to remove any processing chemicals from the film. The fixer (choice 2) follows the rinse bath. The dryer (choice 4) is the final step in the development process.

2. **The correct answer is 1.** Underfiltration may result in diminished radiographic content. Increased object-film distance (choice 2), a patient that is not parallel to the film (choice 3), or a patient that is too thick (choice 4) all may result in diminished radiographic detail or definition.

3. **The correct answer is 3.** A higher grid ratio would indicate that more scatter radiation is absorbed. The higher the grid ratio, the more scatter and primary radiation is absorbed. Choice 1 is incorrect because higher grid ratios require a longer exposure time. Choices 2 and 4 are incorrect because these statements would be true only for lower grid ratios.

4. **The correct answer is 3.** Barium, which is a type of positive contrast media, would appear the whitest on an X-ray because it will absorb the greatest amount of X-rays. Bone (choice 1) absorbs the next highest amount of X-rays and would appear white or light gray. Organs (choice 2) absorb some X-rays and would appear gray or dark gray. Fat (choice 4) absorbs the least amount of X-rays and appears very light gray or translucent on an X-ray.

5. **The correct answer is 1.** A damaged grid may result in black marks on a developed radiograph. Inadequate rinsing (choice 2) may lead to a yellow radiograph because any remaining fixer will oxidize to a yellow powder. Debris in the cassette (choice 3) may lead to white marks or clear areas on the developed radiograph. Low processing solutions

(choice 4) may lead to green areas on the developed radiograph.

6. **The correct answer is 4.** The images generated by PET scans are based on the release of positrons caused by the administration of a radioactive tracer isotope. A CT scan (choice 1) works by absorbing photons released from a patient to create a digital image. An MRI (choice 2) creates images using a magnetic field in which radio frequency signals are transmitted and received. An ultrasound (choice 3) uses sound waves to create digital images.

7. **The correct answer is 2.** Acoustic shadowing occurs when sound is completely reflected or absorbed by an object. Refraction (choice 1) occurs when the direction of the sound beam changes while passing between different mediums. Reverberation (choice 3) occurs when sound is constantly reflected between strong reflectors. Mirror image (choice 4) occurs when an organ is lying adjacent to a reflector on the image.

8. **The correct answer is 1.** Dorsoventral is a directional term that indicates an X-ray beam that enters the animal's back and exits through its abdomen. A caudocranial X-ray enters from the tail end of the animal and exits through the head (choice 2). A dorsopalmar X-ray enters from the dorsal aspect of the forelimb and exits at the palmar aspect (choice 3). A dorsoplantar X-ray enters from the dorsal aspect of the hind limb and exits at the plantar aspect (choice 4).

9. **The correct answer is 2.** Incorrect developer temperature can lead to increased film density if the temperature is too high. Improperly mixed developer solution, contaminated developer solution, and diluted developer solution can all lead to decreased film density, so choices 1, 3, and 4 are incorrect.

10. **The correct answer is 4.** Structure mottle is described as the loss of detail due to phosphor variations in the intensifying screen. Radiographic mottle (choice 1) is described as loss of detail due to the size of the individual silver halide crystals. Penumbra (choice 2) is described as a loss of detail because of geometric unsharpness. Quantum mottle (choice 3) is described as a loss of radiographic detail common with faster screens because of unevenly distributed phosphor crystals within the intensifying screen.

SUMMING IT UP

- Veterinarians use diagnostic imaging to explore their patients' internal health and diagnose conditions that cannot be determined by physical examination alone.

- Veterinary technicians are often responsible for producing diagnostic images using devices like X-ray machines, ultrasounds, MRIs, and others. It's important to know how to use these diagnostic imaging devices correctly so that you can produce high-quality, accurate images for the veterinarian.

- Diagnostic imaging questions on the VTNE may include topics such as X-ray science, the X-ray development process, image quality factors, positioning techniques, safety protocols, digital imaging devices, and more.

- Remember to be familiar with the various tools and supplies that you will need to use for diagnostic imaging procedures. Be familiar with any and all safety protocols associated with the diagnostic imaging procedure being performed.

PART IV

Two Written Exam Practice Tests

ANSWER SHEET PRACTICE TEST 2

1. ① ② ③ ④	41. ① ② ③ ④	81. ① ② ③ ④	121. ① ② ③ ④	161. ① ② ③ ④
2. ① ② ③ ④	42. ① ② ③ ④	82. ① ② ③ ④	122. ① ② ③ ④	162. ① ② ③ ④
3. ① ② ③ ④	43. ① ② ③ ④	83. ① ② ③ ④	123. ① ② ③ ④	163. ① ② ③ ④
4. ① ② ③ ④	44. ① ② ③ ④	84. ① ② ③ ④	124. ① ② ③ ④	164. ① ② ③ ④
5. ① ② ③ ④	45. ① ② ③ ④	85. ① ② ③ ④	125. ① ② ③ ④	165. ① ② ③ ④
6. ① ② ③ ④	46. ① ② ③ ④	86. ① ② ③ ④	126. ① ② ③ ④	166. ① ② ③ ④
7. ① ② ③ ④	47. ① ② ③ ④	87. ① ② ③ ④	127. ① ② ③ ④	167. ① ② ③ ④
8. ① ② ③ ④	48. ① ② ③ ④	88. ① ② ③ ④	128. ① ② ③ ④	168. ① ② ③ ④
9. ① ② ③ ④	49. ① ② ③ ④	89. ① ② ③ ④	129. ① ② ③ ④	169. ① ② ③ ④
10. ① ② ③ ④	50. ① ② ③ ④	90. ① ② ③ ④	130. ① ② ③ ④	170. ① ② ③ ④
11. ① ② ③ ④	51. ① ② ③ ④	91. ① ② ③ ④	131. ① ② ③ ④	171. ① ② ③ ④
12. ① ② ③ ④	52. ① ② ③ ④	92. ① ② ③ ④	132. ① ② ③ ④	172. ① ② ③ ④
13. ① ② ③ ④	53. ① ② ③ ④	93. ① ② ③ ④	133. ① ② ③ ④	173. ① ② ③ ④
14. ① ② ③ ④	54. ① ② ③ ④	94. ① ② ③ ④	134. ① ② ③ ④	174. ① ② ③ ④
15. ① ② ③ ④	55. ① ② ③ ④	95. ① ② ③ ④	135. ① ② ③ ④	175. ① ② ③ ④
16. ① ② ③ ④	56. ① ② ③ ④	96. ① ② ③ ④	136. ① ② ③ ④	176. ① ② ③ ④
17. ① ② ③ ④	57. ① ② ③ ④	97. ① ② ③ ④	137. ① ② ③ ④	177. ① ② ③ ④
18. ① ② ③ ④	58. ① ② ③ ④	98. ① ② ③ ④	138. ① ② ③ ④	178. ① ② ③ ④
19. ① ② ③ ④	59. ① ② ③ ④	99. ① ② ③ ④	139. ① ② ③ ④	179. ① ② ③ ④
20. ① ② ③ ④	60. ① ② ③ ④	100. ① ② ③ ④	140. ① ② ③ ④	180. ① ② ③ ④
21. ① ② ③ ④	61. ① ② ③ ④	101. ① ② ③ ④	141. ① ② ③ ④	181. ① ② ③ ④
22. ① ② ③ ④	62. ① ② ③ ④	102. ① ② ③ ④	142. ① ② ③ ④	182. ① ② ③ ④
23. ① ② ③ ④	63. ① ② ③ ④	103. ① ② ③ ④	143. ① ② ③ ④	183. ① ② ③ ④
24. ① ② ③ ④	64. ① ② ③ ④	104. ① ② ③ ④	144. ① ② ③ ④	184. ① ② ③ ④
25. ① ② ③ ④	65. ① ② ③ ④	105. ① ② ③ ④	145. ① ② ③ ④	185. ① ② ③ ④
26. ① ② ③ ④	66. ① ② ③ ④	106. ① ② ③ ④	146. ① ② ③ ④	186. ① ② ③ ④
27. ① ② ③ ④	67. ① ② ③ ④	107. ① ② ③ ④	147. ① ② ③ ④	187. ① ② ③ ④
28. ① ② ③ ④	68. ① ② ③ ④	108. ① ② ③ ④	148. ① ② ③ ④	188. ① ② ③ ④
29. ① ② ③ ④	69. ① ② ③ ④	109. ① ② ③ ④	149. ① ② ③ ④	189. ① ② ③ ④
30. ① ② ③ ④	70. ① ② ③ ④	110. ① ② ③ ④	150. ① ② ③ ④	190. ① ② ③ ④
31. ① ② ③ ④	71. ① ② ③ ④	111. ① ② ③ ④	151. ① ② ③ ④	191. ① ② ③ ④
32. ① ② ③ ④	72. ① ② ③ ④	112. ① ② ③ ④	152. ① ② ③ ④	192. ① ② ③ ④
33. ① ② ③ ④	73. ① ② ③ ④	113. ① ② ③ ④	153. ① ② ③ ④	193. ① ② ③ ④
34. ① ② ③ ④	74. ① ② ③ ④	114. ① ② ③ ④	154. ① ② ③ ④	194. ① ② ③ ④
35. ① ② ③ ④	75. ① ② ③ ④	115. ① ② ③ ④	155. ① ② ③ ④	195. ① ② ③ ④
36. ① ② ③ ④	76. ① ② ③ ④	116. ① ② ③ ④	156. ① ② ③ ④	196. ① ② ③ ④
37. ① ② ③ ④	77. ① ② ③ ④	117. ① ② ③ ④	157. ① ② ③ ④	197. ① ② ③ ④
38. ① ② ③ ④	78. ① ② ③ ④	118. ① ② ③ ④	158. ① ② ③ ④	198. ① ② ③ ④
39. ① ② ③ ④	79. ① ② ③ ④	119. ① ② ③ ④	159. ① ② ③ ④	199. ① ② ③ ④
40. ① ② ③ ④	80. ① ② ③ ④	120. ① ② ③ ④	160. ① ② ③ ④	200. ① ② ③ ④

Practice Test 2

1. Alpha-2 agonists, used therapeutically, decrease cardiac output in most animals. This decrease is due to:
   1. decreased afterload.
   2. coronary vasoconstriction.
   3. high catecholamine levels.
   4. increased myocardial oxygen consumption.

2. Which of the following is a reason geriatric patients should be scheduled for surgery before young patients?
   1. Young patients become stressed more easily.
   2. Geriatric patients take longer to recover.
   3. Young patients need to eat more often.
   4. Geriatric patients do not have to drink so often.

3. Which teeth are primarily used for cutting, shearing, and holding?
   1. Premolars
   2. Incisors
   3. Molars
   4. Canines

4. Which of the following is a correct statement concerning tissue samples?
   1. Once removed from the animal, tissue immediately starts to die.
   2. The process of autolysis is accelerated by cool temperatures.
   3. Fixing tissues hastens the deterioration of cell membranes.
   4. Tissues for standard histological examination should be frozen.

5. All the following are true of veterinarian-client-patient relationships *except*:
   1. the client and owner of the patient should be skeptical of the veterinarian.
   2. the veterinarian should regularly visit animals in the clinic or in the field.
   3. the client and owner of the patient should be honest with the veterinarian.
   4. the veterinarian should be on-call and available in the event of an emergency.

6. Which of the following is a major disadvantage in performing fluoroscopic studies on animals?
   1. These studies are often expensive, so owners choose not to consent to testing.
   2. These studies' images can be saved in a variety of ways, including videotape.
   3. These studies expose veterinary personnel to radiation.
   4. These studies replace angiographic catheters.

7. Veterinary technicians may use the tape technique to examine an area of skin for all the following *except*:
   1. bacteria.
   2. ringworm.
   3. Malassezia.
   4. surface mites.

8. After surgical equipment is sterilized, it is packaged and stored. Items can become unsterile if they are not stored or handled properly. Which of the following surgical items is still sterile?
   1. The item was stored in a humid area, and the packing is now wet.
   2. A technician pulled back the packing without touching the paper to the instrument.
   3. The item was stored in a pack that was punctured by another instrument.
   4. A technician pulled back the packing and touched the item with his forearm.

9. All the following statements about general toxicology specimens are true *except*:
   1. They should not be washed or submitted to extraneous contamination.
   2. They should be submitted in leak-proof and sterile glass or plastic containers.
   3. They should be collected fresh and then delivered to the lab frozen.
   4. They should not be individually labeled; only the largest containers need labels.

10. Many veterinary clinics do not line kennel floors with newspapers because newspapers are not:
    1. readily available.
    2. easily disposable.
    3. absorbent.
    4. warm.

11. A correct statement regarding amiodarone, a common class III antiarrhythmic agent, is that it:
    1. has a low iodine content.
    2. metabolizes to desethylamiodarone in dogs.
    3. blocks slow-moving sodium channels.
    4. is structurally related to carvedilol.

12. A correct statement regarding the use of atracurium as a muscle paralytic is it:
    1. does not cause a release of histamine.
    2. decreases intraocular pressure.
    3. does not cause sympathetic stimulation.
    4. is immediately effective.

13. Technicians may occasionally care for cats experiencing Key-Gaskell Syndrome. All the following statements are true regarding this condition *except* it:
    1. is also known as feline dysautonomia.
    2. affects the autonomic nervous system.
    3. tends to appear in cats aged 3 years or older.
    4. affects more cats on the West Coast than the East Coast.

14. In a generally healthy patient, an anesthetic that is administered intravenously will *most likely* take effect within a few:
    1. seconds.
    2. minutes.
    3. hours.
    4. days.

15. Veterinary medical teams wish to meet four goals when anesthetizing a patient for ophthalmic surgery. These include all the following *except* to:
    1. provide a mobile eye.
    2. provide a pain-free recovery.
    3. support cardiopulmonary function.
    4. avoid increases in intraocular pressure.

16. A correct statement concerning a Michel's trephine is it is:
    1. most often used for bone biopsies.
    2. able to cut a square hole through bone.
    3. only available in one diameter.
    4. battery or electric-power operated.

17. Which of the following urine preservatives is used for biochemical analyses of urea, ammonia, calcium, nitrogen, and uric acid in animals?
    1. Toluene
    2. Acetic acid
    3. Chloroform
    4. Hydrochloric acid

18. Which of the following types of anticestodal drugs is used to eliminate the presence of most species of tapeworms except *Spirometra mansonoides* and *Diphyllobothrium erinacei* in dogs and cats?
    1. Praziquantel
    2. Niclosamide
    3. Bunamidine
    4. Albendazole

19. A veterinary technician receives a frantic call from a pet owner. From what the owner says, the technician concludes the owner's dog has consciously collapsed with dyspnea. In which of the following categories of emergency should the technician place the patient?
    1. Nonemergency
    2. Minor
    3. Serious
    4. Life threatening

20. During which of the stages of anesthesia does the patient react to external stimulus with a struggling reflex?
    1. Stage 1
    2. Stage 2
    3. Stage 3
    4. Stage 4

21. Which of the following is a correct statement regarding the collection of animal feces?
    1. Better results come from feces collected from the ground or litter box than fresh feces.
    2. It is best to collect feces before collecting urine to avoid contaminating the urine.
    3. Feces collection usually requires restraining the animal so the process is uninterrupted.
    4. If it is difficult to collect the feces, it should be forced out of the animal using lubricant.

22. Thiacetarsamide sodium is most frequently used as treatment for:
    1. hookworms.
    2. heartworms.
    3. roundworms.
    4. tapeworms.

23. Surgeons can use all the following types of powered equipment in an operating room *except* a/an:
    1. oscillating saw.
    2. pneumatic drill.
    3. electric drill.
    4. rotary saw.

24. When performing colorimetric biological determinations, veterinary technicians may notice an abnormal change in the color of plasma and serum due to high chromatin levels. When performing this test on a grazing animal, such as a dairy cow, technicians may notice serum and plasma colored:
    1. red.
    2. green.
    3. yellow.
    4. blue.

25. Which of the following muscles should veterinary technicians avoid during intramuscular injections?
    1. Quadriceps group
    2. Gluteal muscles
    3. Triceps muscles
    4. Lumbodorsal muscles

26. Which of the following statements is true about patients undergoing anesthesia?
    1. Very young patients should not fast for long before anesthesia because they could become hypoglycemic.
    2. A dog in good health cannot consume food or water for 12 hours before undergoing surgery.
    3. Patients undergoing joint surgeries generally have to fast longer than patients undergoing abdominal surgeries.
    4. Most normal, healthy patient have to fast for about 4 hours before they undergo surgery.

27. Which of the following instruments would a surgeon use for ligation of stumps or pedicles?
    1. Halsted mosquito hemostatic forceps
    2. Rochester-Carmalt hemostatic forceps
    3. Doyen intestinal forceps
    4. Babock intestinal forceps

28. Which of the following is a correct statement regarding subcutaneous injections?
    1. The effects are felt 15–20 minutes after the injection.
    2. This area contains a small supply of blood vessels.
    3. The area below the skin's surface has many nerves.
    4. Only nonirritant drugs should be administered this way.

29. Within which part of an image-intensified fluoroscopic system are X-rays converted into visible light photons?
    1. Output fluorescent screen
    2. Image intensifier tube
    3. Electrostatic lenses
    4. Fluoroscopic tube

30. Which of the following anesthesia drugs is *most often* injected?
    1. Isoflurane
    2. Ether
    3. Halothane
    4. Morphine

31. A correct statement regarding a common dental instrument called a *curette* is:
    1. it has two blades and one cutting edge.
    2. it is used to remove subgigival calculus.
    3. it cannot be used for removal of soft tissue diseases.
    4. its cutting edges cannot be used on the back of the tooth.

32. While conducting wildlife research, scientists may discover an animal, such as a wild bird, that needs immediate medical attention. Which of the following procedures would a surgeon be *least likely* to perform on a wild animal?
    1. Laparotomy
    2. Flight restraint
    3. Sterilization
    4. Dental prophylaxis

33. Hemolysis occurs when red blood cells break and release their contents into blood serum or plasma. All the following are causes of in vitro hemolysis *except*:
    1. osmotic pressure.
    2. the size of the needle.
    3. the separation of plasma.
    4. vigorous shaking of samples.

34. Which of the following is true about a Robert Jones bandage?
    1. The bandage can last for up to a month.
    2. The bandage should always include the toes.
    3. The bandage contains traction tape to decrease slippage.
    4. The bandage does not require a large quantity of cotton wool.

35. The darkest, or least opaque, parts of an X-ray indicate the presence of:
    1. gas.
    2. muscle.
    3. bone.
    4. mineral.

36. When administering an anesthetic to a horse intravenously, technicians inject the anesthetic into the:
    1. jugular vein.
    2. cephalic vein.
    3. saphenous vein.
    4. mesenteric vein.

37. The use of piperazine, an antinematodal agent, is recommended in all the following *except*:
    1. cats.
    2. dogs.
    3. pigs.
    4. cattle.

38. Technicians must often administer medications, such as a hypodermic injection, to patients. When administering a hypodermic injection, a technician may inject the drug using all the following routes *except*:
    1. subcutaneous.
    2. intramuscular.
    3. intravenous.
    4. epidural.

39. If an adult bovine has 32 teeth, what is the animal's dental formula?
    1. I0/6 C1/2 P3/6
    2. I6/6 C1/2 P3-4/3 M3/3
    3. I0/6 C0/2 P6/6 M6/6
    4. I3/6 C1/2 P4/8 M3/6

40. A correct statement regarding needle holders is:
    1. they are not involved in metal-to-metal contact.
    2. as they wear, they become blunt or dull.
    3. they are easily replaceable.
    4. large needle holders are required for delicate sutures.

41. Generally, urine samples are collected and stored in:
    1. glass Vacutainers.
    2. plastic Petri dishes.
    3. plastic sample bottles.
    4. glass vials.

42. Which of the following dressings retains moisture within the wound?
    1. Dry dressings
    2. Occlusive dressings
    3. Hemostatic dressings
    4. Impregnated gauze dressings

43. When collecting cerebrospinal fluid, the area of the spine that veterinary technicians *most* frequently tap is the:
    1. axis.
    2. atlas.
    3. occipital bone.
    4. atlanto-occipital joint.

44. When performing a venous portography, technicians inject positive contrast media into the spleen or the:
    1. mesenteric vein.
    2. cephalic vein.
    3. saphenous vein.
    4. jugular vein.

45. Procedures on bigger animals, such as horses or cows, may occur either in the field or in a clinic. Which of the following methods of monitoring a larger animal's status would a veterinary technician *least likely* use while in the field?
    1. Personal observation
    2. Pulse palpitation
    3. A stethoscope
    4. Blood pressure monitoring

46. An example of a tricyclic antidepressant used in veterinary medicine is:
    1. tofranil.
    2. ativan.
    3. valium.
    4. risperdal.

47. Which of the following first-aid situations requires immediate medical attention for a member of a veterinary medical team?
    1. Ingestion of chemical agents
    2. Skin contact with chemical agents
    3. Eye contact with biological agents
    4. Wounds from sharp biological agents

48. When drawing blood from small animals such as dogs and cats, the vein of choice is generally the:
    1. cephalic.
    2. jugular.
    3. renal.
    4. saphenous.

49. Saffan, a steroid anesthetic, is a mixture of alphaxalone and alphadolone. Technicians intravenously inject a dose of 3–6 mg/kg in:
    1. cats.
    2. dogs.
    3. birds.
    4. rabbits.

50. Emesis may be recommended in all the following cases *except* to:
    1. empty the stomach before surgery.
    2. eliminate a toxin.

3. remove a small toy.
4. eradicate corrosive poisoning.

51. An ideal operating room has:
    1. one door.
    2. two doors.
    3. three doors.
    4. four doors.

52. While horses awaiting surgery can drink water up to 1 hour before the procedure, they must fast for:
    1. 6 hours.
    2. 10 hours.
    3. 12 hours.
    4. 14 hours.

53. Which of the following agents is considered an inappropriate antiseptic due to its caustic nature?
    1. Witch hazel
    2. Bacitracin zinc
    3. Formaldehyde
    4. Polymyxin B sulfate

54. In the lab, a technician accidentally spills biological agents on the skin exposed between his wrists and his lab coat. He knows the situation requires immediate first aid, and he performs all the following emergency actions *except*:
    1. rinsing with water.
    2. wiping with antiseptic cloths.
    3. lathering with soap.
    4. scrubbing with a sponge.

55. Technicians often pay special attention to recumbent animals, or those who must remain lying down for recovery. These animals receive extra padding in their beds, are turned every 2–4 hours, and receive physiotherapy. Physiotherapy may include all the following *except*:
    1. coupage.
    2. massage.
    3. ice baths.
    4. hydrotherapy.

56. A veterinarian orders an X-ray in which a dog must be positioned so that it is lying on its right side. The technician will use a horizontal X-ray beam to capture an image of the dog's chest. What is the name of this position?
    1. Ventrodorsal projection
    2. Cranial caudal projection
    3. Right lateral projection
    4. Right-left lateral recumbent projection

57. All the following are true statements concerning the use of anesthesia on horses *except*:
    1. local anesthetics are often used as diagnostic tools.
    2. all procedures are completed while the horses lay on their sides.
    3. general anesthetics are used for procedures such as cheek teeth removal.
    4. anesthetics create a higher level of safety for handlers and technicians.

58. When Beta-blockers are administered intravenously to dogs, veterinary technicians should closely monitor:
    1. blood pressure and electrocardiograms.
    2. X-rays and electrocardiograms.
    3. blood pressure and breathing sounds.
    4. bleeding and breath sounds.

59. While preparing for surgery, surgeons and veterinary technicians should thoroughly wash their hands and forearms. Hands and forearms should be exposed to antiseptic scrubs for no less than:
    1. 30 seconds.
    2. 1 minute.
    3. 90 seconds.
    4. 2 minutes.

60. While working in the lab, a veterinary technician notices a gray Vacutainer with a yellow collecting pot on the counter. The Vacutainer the technician is looking at contains the anticoagulant:
    1. heparin.
    2. EDTA.
    3. oxalate fluoride.
    4. sodium citrate.

61. All the following materials are often used to pad bandages *except*:
    1. foam.
    2. Soft Ban.
    3. Bubble Wrap.
    4. cotton wool.

62. Which of the following drugs is an opioid?
    1. Ketoprofen
    2. Morphine
    3. Aspirin
    4. Lidocaine

63. Which of the following steps should a veterinary technician complete first when bandaging an animal's ear?
    1. Fold the ear back onto a pad of cotton wool.
    2. Apply a conforming bandage over the ear and under the chin.
    3. Apply a dry dressing and place another pad of cotton wool over the ear.
    4. Cover the bandage with adhesive tape.

64. Which of the following patients should be monitored the closest during general anesthesia?
    1. A dog with a heart rate 100 beats per minute
    2. A dog that is obese
    3. A cat with a heart rate of 150 beats per minute
    4. A cat with a normal weight

65. Studies in 2006 found that the use of acepromazine, an antipsychotic drug, often increases the risk of seizures in all these animals *except*:
    1. cats.
    2. squirrels.
    3. dogs.
    4. bats.

66. A correct statement concerning the alcohols used as disinfectants or antiseptics before, during, or after surgeries is they:
    1. are drying agents.
    2. have a weak defatting effect.
    3. do not require the presence of water.
    4. are not effective in the first two minutes of application.

67. The teeth of carnivores and herbivores differ due to the various materials they eat. Which of the following parts are common in herbivore teeth but *not* common in carnivore teeth?
    1. Dentin
    2. Pulp cavity
    3. Cementum
    4. Infundibulum

68. While working in the lab, a technician witnesses a fellow coworker fumble with a bottle before it falls to the floor and breaks. Upon closer inspection, the technician realizes that the liquid is highly flammable. To clean a spill containing flammable liquid, the technician needs all the following materials *except*:
1. sand.
2. water.
3. autoclave.
4. detergent.

69. A veterinarian meets with a new client whose Yorkshire terrier has a few dog shows scheduled for the future. The Yorkshire terrier has developed an abnormal set of eyelashes, and the owner has noticed that the dog's eyes have been tearing and inflamed. The veterinarian diagnoses the dog with a genetic defect called distichia, which can cause scarring. What should the veterinarian do?
1. The veterinarian should refuse to complete the surgery because it is unethical to cure genetic defects in show dogs.
2. The veterinarian should agree to perform the surgery, but he/she must tell the owner she can no longer show or breed the dog.
3. The veterinarian should refuse to perform the surgery because it is the first time he/she has met the owner or the dog.
4. The veterinarian should agree to perform the surgery but should charge the owner a higher price for treating a show dog.

70. Based on observations of a cat's limited and painful movements, a veterinarian recommends and the cat's owners agree to an examination in which the veterinarian can achieve a closer look at the cat's spinal cord. Which of the following tests is the veterinarian recommending?
1. Celiography
2. Myelography
3. Angiography
4. Epidurography

71. Which of the following is a correct statement concerning a technician's attempt to maintain an animal's mental stimulation and morale?
1. Toys from home are not allowed in the kennel.
2. Visits by the owner are not advisable.

3. The animal's name should be used frequently.
4. Regular grooming is not necessary.

72. All the following statements regarding the use of a local anesthetic as an adjunct to surgical anesthesia are true *except*:
1. the combined technique is useful in high-risk surgeries.
2. the local technique affects cardiopulmonary function.
3. animals recover consciousness rapidly.
4. the surgical sites remain pain free.

73. You are about to perform an orogastric intubation on a large, 24-pound dog. What size stomach tube would be *most* appropriate for use in this scenario?
1. 12 French
2. 14 French
3. 16 French
4. 18 French

74. An animal is in anesthesia Stage 3. Which of the following signs would indicate the patient is in plane III?
1. Deep and regular respirations
2. Fixed and centrally rotated eyeballs
3. Pale mucus membranes
4. Half thoracic and half abdominal respiration

75. When prepping a patient for surgery, veterinary technicians use antiseptics that are split into three different categories. Antiseptics are placed in the second category if they possess the ability to prevent recontamination of the skin up to six hours. The second category measures the antiseptic's:
1. immediate efficacy.
2. prolonged usefulness.
3. persistent microbial effectiveness.
4. residual action.

76. All the following are true statements about teeth *except*:
1. teeth are not dead structures.
2. teeth have their own nerve supply.
3. teeth have their own blood vessels.
4. teeth are not susceptible to pain.

77. Which of the following is the term most frequently used to refer to the input and output of body water over a specific period of time?
    1. Water shed
    2. Water monitoring
    3. Water turnover
    4. Water quality

78. Colorimetry is a measurement of:
    1. color.
    2. sound.
    3. light.
    4. waves.

79. A correct statement regarding feeding an animal in recovery is that the food should be:
    1. easy to digest.
    2. served fresh and cold.
    3. left out for when the animal is hungry.
    4. placed in an area that requires the animal to move to it.

80. Upper gastrointestinal studies (UGIs) allow for assessment of the:
    1. kidneys and small intestine.
    2. liver and large intestine.
    3. stomach and small intestine.
    4. colon and large intestine.

81. One easy way to tell if a patient is unsuited for anesthesia is to:
    1. examine the patient's eating habits.
    2. take the patient for a walk.
    3. observe the patient while he or she sleeps.
    4. test the patient's urine and fecal matter.

82. Martin, a veterinary technician, sees another technician drop a vial of blood on the floor. The coworker cleans the spill and reports it to her supervisor. After witnessing the incident Martin should:
    1. report the incident to the American Veterinary Medical Association because the worker was negligent.
    2. not report the incident to the American Veterinary Medical Association because the worker took the proper steps after the spill.

    3. report the incident to the American Veterinary Medical Association because the worker should have called the patient's owner about the spill.
    4. not report the incident to the American Veterinary Medical Association because the worker was not a veterinarian.

83. A veterinarian schedules an operation on a 4-month-old kitten. Before the operation, the kitten must be bathed and must fast for no longer than:
    1. 4 hours.
    2. 6 hours.
    3. 8 hours.
    4. 12 hours.

84. In dogs, which teeth are called the *carnassial teeth*?
    1. First molar in the lower arcade and fourth premolar in the upper arcade
    2. Second molar in the lower arcade and third premolar in the upper arcade
    3. Third molar in the lower arcade and first premolar in the upper arcade
    4. Fourth molar in the lower arcade and second premolar in the upper arcade

85. After you have finished using a compound microscope, what is the last step you must complete before covering it?
    1. Lower the stage.
    2. Turn off the light.
    3. Turn down the rheostat.
    4. Clean the oil immersion lens.

86. Newborn animals are often poikilothermic and placed in incubators. Ideally, incubator temperatures should be set at:
    1. 78–83°F.
    2. 86–91°F.
    3. 95–100°F.
    4. 101–106°F.

87. All the following are true about healing using granulation tissue *except*:
    1. the edges of the wound stay close together.
    2. the wound often becomes infected.
    3. healing can take weeks to months.
    4. scarring is often extensive.

88. Rhinography is a contrast study of the:
1. nasal cavity.
2. cranial cavity.
3. pelvic cavity.
4. thoracic cavity.

89. Which of the following is true about an animal that is treated with ketamine?
1. Its pupils constrict.
2. Its eyes remain closed.
3. Its cranial nerve reflexes are more depressed.
4. Its protective airway reflexes are maintained.

90. A correct statement regarding the identifying traits of canine teeth is that they:
1. are known as "cheek" teeth.
2. have flat, occlusal surfaces.
3. may appear as tusks in some species.
4. have multiple sharp points in carnivores.

91. Which anesthetic can cause fetal depression when used?
1. Halothane
2. Thiopental
3. Sevoflurane
4. Etomidate

92. A puppy undergoing surgery is monitored with pulse oximeter. Which of the following describes the function of a pulse oximeter?
1. Monitors the puppy's direct systolic and diastolic blood pressure
2. Charts the puppy's pulse rate and oxygen levels in the blood
3. Monitors the puppy's pulse rate and pulse rhythm
4. Charts the puppy's respiratory air movement

93. Of the following, the microorganism that is *most* resistant to disinfectant killing is:
1. fungi.
2. vegetative bacteria.
3. lipid-coated viruses.
4. bacterial endospores.

94. Which of the following types of blocking drugs is often administered before anesthesia to prevent the stimulation of visceral tissues?
1. Beta
2. Neuromuscular
3. Autonomic
4. Acid

95. After completing an operation on a dog, you notice one of the dog's pupils is bigger than the other one. This condition is called:
1. anisocoria.
2. cherry eye.
3. entropion.
4. glaucoma.

96. A healthy dog or cat may exhibit the following signs *except*:
1. clear eyes free of discharge.
2. clean and odor-free ears.
3. free limb movement.
4. white mucous membranes.

97. Significant weight loss increases surgical risks in animals. The majority of animals are at risk of death or postoperative complications if weight loss has reached:
1. 5% of body weight.
2. 10% of body weight.
3. 15 % of body weight.
4. 20% of body weight.

98. How many teeth are typically in an adult dog's mouth?
1. 26
2. 28
3. 30
4. 42

99. Which part of a compound microscope holds the slide?
1. Stage
2. Rotating turret
3. Optical tube
4. Substage condenser

100. An 11-year-old cat is brought to the veterinary office for the sixth time in two months for a urinary tract infection. The veterinarian orders an X-ray with a dye injected into the animal's veins to examine the kidneys, ureters, and urinary bladder. Which of the following is the name for this type of test?

1. Urohydropropulsion
2. Intravenous pyelogram
3. CAT scan
4. Perineal urethrostomy

101. Veterinary patients are placed in five categories of risk assessment determined by the American Society of Anesthesiologists. A patient with a mild systemic disease would be placed in:

1. Class 1.
2. Class 2.
3. Class 3.
4. Class 4.

102. If a veterinary technician is attempting to measure the pulse in a dog's or cat's tail, he or she is monitoring the:

1. femoral artery.
2. digital artery.
3. coccygeal artery.
4. lingual artery.

103. Resorptive lesions are found primarily in which of the following animals?

1. Cats
2. Lizards
3. Cattle
4. Horses

104. Before an 8-year-old dog undergoes surgery, a veterinary technician completes a physical examination. During the examination of the dog's respiratory system, the technician notices percussive sounds with high resonance. This condition is consistent with:

1. airway secretion.
2. respiratory disease.
3. lung consolidation.
4. pneumothorax.

105. A technician is treating a patient experiencing a change in appetite. Rather than a loss of interest in food, the owner says it seems as though her dog is never satisfied and is always looking for more to eat. The technician decides that the dog is experiencing:

1. pica.
2. polyuria.
3. coprophagia.
4. voracious appetite.

106. Of the following animals, which is *most likely* to attack when taken from their home and placed in an unfamiliar environment, such as a veterinary clinic?

1. Cats
2. Dogs
3. Birds
4. Ferrets

107. Which of the following uses a magnetic field to produce images of internal organs and tissues?

1. X-ray
2. MRI
3. CAT scan
4. Biopsy

108. Touching the surface of the patient's eye tests which of the following reflexes during anesthesia?

1. Palpebral
2. Corneal
3. Pupillary
4. Withdrawal

109. Which of the following can be used to treat Pacheco's disease in birds?

1. Fluconazole
2. Metronidazole
3. Acyclovir
4. Oseltamivir

110. Shock is a serious risk in pre-, intra-, and postsurgical environments. No matter the initial cause, the inciting event of shock is always:

1. tachycardia.
2. circulatory collapse.
3. decrease in blood flow.
4. dehydration.

111. The dental formula for an adult cat is:

1. i6/6 c2/2 p6/6.
2. I6/6 C2/2 P 8/8 M6/6.
3. i6/6 c2/2 p6/4.
4. I6/6 C2/2 P6/4 M2/2.

112. All the following animals lack the ability to regurgitate *except*:
    1. rats.
    2. rabbits.
    3. horses.
    4. ferrets.

113. When cleaning glassware in a laboratory, you must first soak the dirty glassware in disinfectant. Immediately after scrubbing debris or surface material off the glass, you should:
    1. rinse it thoroughly in distilled water.
    2. soak it in detergent or an ultrasonic bath.
    3. allow the excess liquids to drain.
    4. allow it to air dry or place it in a drying oven.

114. Feulgen stain is used to examine which of the following?
    1. Lipids
    2. Connective tissue
    3. Chromosomes
    4. Bacteria

115. A technician can reduce the stress levels of her patients by:
    1. creating loud noises that are comforting to animals away from home.
    2. making eye contact with all canines and speaking softly to them.
    3. placing cats in cages where they cannot be seen by other animals.
    4. allowing animals to urinate or defecate in their cages or stalls.

116. Which of the following is the average gestation period for sheep?
    1. 103 days
    2. 121 days
    3. 147 days
    4. 179 days

117. The optimum conditions for reading a radiograph include:
    1. a brightly lit room.
    2. dim lighting.
    3. glossy films.
    4. little to no glare.

118. The maximum weight of a surgical instrument pack being placed into an autoclave should be:
    1. 4.5 kg.
    2. 5.0 kg.
    3. 5.5 kg.
    4. 6.0 kg.

119. The outermost layer of an animal's tooth is the:
    1. apex.
    2. dentin.
    3. enamel.
    4. pulp.

120. A correct statement regarding universal sterile containers is that they are:
    1. large bottles.
    2. narrow-mouthed bottles.
    3. made of either plastic or glass.
    4. often designed to hold more than 300 ml of fluid.

121. Polydipsia is a symptom of which of the following conditions?
    1. Nephritis
    2. Cystic calculi
    3. Prostatic enlargement
    4. Obstruction of the urinary tract

122. After administering norepinephrine, extreme vasoconstriction occurs. This means peripheral resistance:
    1. increases and blood flow increases.
    2. decreases and blood flow decreases.
    3. increases and blood flow decreases.
    4. decreases and blood flow increases.

123. A correct statement regarding isoproterenol is that this myocardial stimulant:
    1. is dependent on alterations in venous returns.
    2. increases the strength of contractile forces and accelerates heart rate.
    3. is 30–40 times more active in the heart than epinephrine.
    4. decreases the rate of pressure changes in the ventricular chambers.

124. Ideal operating room conditions include a temperature of approximately:
1. 60°F and humidity of approximately 50%.
2. 70°F and humidity of approximately 60%.
3. 70°F and humidity of approximately 50%.
4. 50°F and humidity of approximately 70%.

125. An ideal antiseptic:
1. has high toxicity.
2. has low penetrability.
3. performs a narrow spectrum of activity.
4. causes little skin irritation or interference.

126. A veterinary technician treats a dog diagnosed with parvovirus. The technician tells the dog's owner to perform surface disinfection on cages, carpets, couches, and other areas in the owner's home. The technician also tells the owner to clean the dog's toys and food and water bowls by placing these smaller objects in a tub of disinfectant for a specific period of time. This process is often referred to as:
1. cold sterilization.
2. immersion disinfection.
3. heat-pressure sterilization.
4. physical disinfection.

127. Before deciding whether a surgery is necessary, veterinarians perform physical examinations. Within the first few seconds of the exam, veterinarians examine all the following *except* the animal's:
1. attitude.
2. walk.
3. nutritional status.
4. rate of respiration.

128. All of these statements are true about microscopes *except*:
1. oil must be cleaned from the oil immersion lens before it dries.
2. to find the true magnification, multiply the objective magnification by the ocular magnification.
3. the base of the microscope should be at least 10 cm away from a table's edge.
4. when using the coarse focus, you should adjust the knobs very quickly to find the right focus.

129. A cat has been in the care of a technician for two days. Over those two days, the technician has noticed the cat has vomited multiple times. Between bouts of vomiting, the cat appears to be free of symptoms. The technician notes a lack of blood, feces, and bile in the vomit. Which of the following types of vomiting is the cat experiencing?
1. Bilious vomiting
2. Cyclic vomiting
3. Projectile vomiting
4. Stercoraceous vomiting

130. A technician needs to evaluate bladder wall integrity and bladder position in a young dog. Which of the following cystography contrast studies should the technician perform?
1. Positive contrast cystography
2. Negative contrast cystography
3. Double contrast cystography
4. Pneumocystography

131. Many drugs for animals, in combination with behavioral modification therapies, are used to:
1. increase arousal.
2. decrease compulsivity.
3. increase excitability.
4. decrease behavioral calming.

132. Which of the following organs is responsible for metabolizing anesthetic drugs and producing plasma proteins and coagulation factors?
1. Lungs
2. Liver
3. Heart
4. Kidneys

133. The presence of blood in an animal's urine is called:
1. anuria.
2. dysuria.
3. oliguria.
4. hematuria.

134. A common side effect of phenothiazines is a/an:
1. decrease in achieving arousal.
2. increase in spontaneous motor activity.
3. decrease in coordinated motor responses.
4. increase in extrapyramidal symptoms.

135. The pelvic limb swing is an immobilizer that:
1. allows the hind legs to bear weight but prevents the leg muscles from moving.
2. prohibits the hind legs from bearing weight but allows movement of the joints.
3. encases the entire hind or front leg and does not allow muscle or joint movement.
4. prohibits the front legs from bearing weight and relieves tension in the tendons.

136. A veterinary technician is assisting in the bandaging of a dog's tail. The bandage the technician is helping to apply is *most likely* a:
1. white open wove bandage.
2. cohesive bandage.
3. tubular bandage.
4. crepe bandage.

137. Which of these veterinary technicians is acting unethically?
1. Samantha states on a resume that she is a current member of an organization that she stopped paying dues to last year.
2. Ethan asks to rearrange his work schedule to accommodate taking continuing education classes.
3. Gerard discloses information about one of the patients at his clinic after receiving a request from a public health organization.
4. Natasha discusses possible treatments options for one of her patients with another technician at her clinic.

138. Urinary catheterization includes the placement of a small, plastic tube into an animal's bladder via its urethra. Which of the following animals rarely receive catheterization?
1. Female cats
2. Male dogs
3. Female pigs
4. Male horses

139. Which of the following suture materials generally takes the longest to absorb?
1. Polyglactin 910
2. Polyglycolic acid
3. Polydioxanone
4. Poliglecaprone 25

140. The part of the microscope that connects the base and stage is the:
1. arm.
2. rheostat.
3. illuminator.
4. condenser.

141. In an ideal situation, a technician would take an animal's temperature via the patient's:
1. axilla.
2. rectum.
3. mouth.
4. ear canal.

142. Pyrexia is caused by the following *except*:
1. infection.
2. convulsions.
3. hypothermia.
4. excitement.

143. Many behavioral drugs are water-soluble salts. This means these drugs allow for:
1. slow dissolution in the gastrointestinal tract and good permeability in the intestine.
2. rapid dissolution in the gastrointestinal tract and good permeability in the intestine.
3. rapid dissolution in the gastrointestinal tract and poor permeability in the intestine.
4. slow dissolution in the gastrointestinal tract and poor permeability in the intestine.

144. A veterinary technician travels to a farm to assess a horse that has a broken leg. The technician notices that nerve and blood vessel damage is present at the sight of the fracture. What type of fracture has occurred?
1. Incomplete fracture
2. Simple fracture
3. Complicated fracture
4. Multiple fracture

145. Ultrasounds have reduced or eliminated the need for:
1. X-rays.
2. radiographic exams.
3. computed tomographies.
4. magnetic resonance imaging.

146. Which of the following is a common side effect of general anesthesia?
1. Low body temperature
2. Reduced body weight
3. Infection
4. Hemorrhaging

147. A correct statement regarding general aminoglycosides is that these molecules have:
1. poor solubility in water.
2. excellent lipid solubility.
3. thermodynamic stability.
4. weights ranging from 100–200 g/mol.

148. If not immediately used, serum or plasma should be stored at:
1. –20°F.
2. –4°F.
3. 15°F.
4. 32°F.

149. A correct statement regarding a cryptorchidism is that it involves the:
1. amputation of a horse's leg.
2. extraction of a horse's testicle.
3. removal of a tumor in a horse.
4. resetting of a horse's broken bone.

150. Which of the following combinations of instruments would a veterinary technician use to trim a rabbit's cheek teeth?
1. Spatula and molar luxator
2. Molar cutters and diamond burr
3. Soft tissue protector and cheek dilator
4. Mouth gag and extraction forceps

151. A correct statement regarding the performance of skin scrapes is that:
1. one goal is to achieve petechial bleeding.
2. skin is scraped until the hypodermis layer is reached.
3. if the sample is going to a lab, the scalpel is not included.
4. it doesn't involve squeezing the skin because the bacteria has already surfaced.

152. A correct statement regarding consulting veterinarians is:
1. consulting veterinarians charge higher fees than attending consultants for their services.
2. consulting veterinarians typically offer their opinions of physical exams and observation of animal behavior.
3. when a consulting veterinarian is called in, he or she is in charge of the veterinarian-client-patient relationship.
4. if a visit to the patient is necessary, consulting veterinarians assess the patient in the presence of the attending veterinarian.

153. All the following statements are true about veterinary medical records *except*:
1. records must comply with state and federal standards.
2. the information in medical records is considered confidential.
3. technicians cannot provide copies of records to clients without a court order.
4. medical records are considered pieces of property belonging to the clinic/practice.

154. If a technician wished to mathematically construct a computerized, cross-sectional image of a cat's brain through measurements received from X-ray transmissions, he or she would recommend that the owner consent to a/an:
1. CT.
2. MRI.
3. UGI.
4. X-ray.

155. The drug epinephrine can be given to patients on anesthesia to make the anesthetic work for:
1. more time by increasing blood flow.
2. less time by increasing blood flow.
3. more time by decreasing blood flow.
4. less time by decreasing blood flow.

156. The amount of total body water elimination due to insensible losses each day in healthy, yet inactive animals residing in a thermo neutral environment is approximately:
1. 5–15 ml/kg.
2. 15–30 ml/kg.
3. 25–40 ml/kg.
4. 35–50 ml/kg.

157. A veterinarian has scheduled an operation in which he will make an incision in a snake's abdomen. This procedure is called:
    1. celiotomy.
    2. lobotomy.
    3. cystotomy.
    4. nephrectomy.

158. It is rare to find a lizard with teeth on its:
    1. palate.
    2. maxilla.
    3. dentary.
    4. premaxilla.

159. Which of the following antiseptics or disinfectants has the ability to preserve tissue samples by hardening, or "fixing," them?
    1. Bleach
    2. Formalin
    3. Triclosan
    4. Glutaraldehyde

160. When caring postoperatively for a patient that had anesthesia, it's important to take special care when bandaging the:
    1. joints.
    2. head.
    3. legs.
    4. paws.

161. A correct statement regarding the use of buspirone in cats is that it:
    1. produces immediate behavioral effects.
    2. impairs memory or psychomotor skills.
    3. regulates states of high arousal.
    4. induces a panic-like state.

162. During surgery, veterinary surgical teams follow aseptic techniques. One of these aseptic techniques is to keep talking to a minimum. Why is refraining from talking an aseptic technique?
    1. Talking may bother the patient that is undergoing surgery.
    2. Talking can break surgeons' concentration, causing them to make mistakes.
    3. Talking releases bacteria in the air, making the operating room less sterile.
    4. Talking could distract members of the surgical team.

163. Veterinary technicians recommend that pet owners brush their pets' teeth at least once a month. If a domestic animal experiences an extreme buildup of plaque or tartar, all the following events will likely occur *except*:
    1. the animal's gums will be red, swollen, and sore.
    2. the animal will develop duplicated canine teeth.
    3. the animal's oral bacteria will enter the bloodstream.
    4. the animal will experience tooth and bone loss.

164. Cats thrive in environments where the temperature is at least:
    1. 50°F.
    2. 60°F.
    3. 70°F.
    4. 80°F.

165. For which group of patients might hypothermia (the lowering of body temperature) be used as a form of anesthesia?
    1. Patients undergoing cardiovascular surgery
    2. Patients undergoing dental surgery
    3. Patients undergoing ophthalmological surgery
    4. Patients undergoing joint surgery

166. Which of the following SSRIs is used to treat dogs that experience dominance-related aggression, inter-dog aggression, or acral lick dermatitis?
    1. Dapoxetine
    2. Fluoxetine
    3. Zimelidine
    4. Indalpine

167. When preparing for surgery, which of the following actions should a veterinary technician perform first?
    1. Put on a cap and mask
    2. Change into a scrub suit
    3. Scrub for surgery
    4. Put on sterile gloves

168. When working with anesthetics, technicians may accidentally expose themselves to the chemical gases or injections they're administering. To avoid self-exposure, technicians can do all the following *except*:
1. empty the rebreathing bag by detaching the bag from the cylinder.
2. place vaporizers outside the operating area when possible.
3. regularly check circuits for leaks.
4. use scavenging systems.

169. The *most* important reason to keep the prophy cup moving while polishing teeth is to:
1. reach as much of each tooth as possible.
2. avoid heating the tooth.
3. remove as much plaque and stain as possible.
4. minimize the pressure required to flare the cup.

170. Synovial fluid is collected through a process called:
1. athrocentesis.
2. thoracocentesis.
3. abdominocentesis.
4. pericardiocentesis.

171. When a technician must handle, or restrain, a dog, he or she should first make the animal feel comfortable. To do this, the technician *must*:
1. make eye contact with the dog.
2. crouch down in front of the dog.
3. sit on the ground in front of the dog.
4. talk to the dog in an excited, high voice.

172. When an animal experiences shock, its urinary patterns may be altered. Of the following, which is *most likely* to occur in an animal that has recently been in shock?
1. Anuria
2. Dysuria
3. Polyuria
4. Polydipsia

173. Which of the following complications are brachycephalic dogs *most likely* to have during anesthesia?
1. Hypothermia
2. Cardiomyopathy
3. Airway blockages
4. Spinal instability

174. After a surgery, animals' wounds should be free of dead space, which can cause bacterial growth. All the following are ways to reduce dead space around wounds *except*:
1. compression bandages
2. drainage
3. Robert Jones bandage
4. splints

175. Technicians perform abdominocentesis to detect an increase in the volume of:
1. synovial fluid.
2. thoracic fluid.
3. peritoneal fluid.
4. cerebrospinal fluid.

176. All the following statements are true about stainless steel cages *except*:
1. they are easy to clean.
2. they are indestructible.
3. they are safe for most animals.
4. they are relatively inexpensive.

177. Which of the following is a nonsteroidal anti-inflammatory drug (NSAID)?
1. Morphine
2. Fentanyl
3. Ketoprofen
4. Butorphanol

178. Following most biopsies, the majority of tissue samples for histopathology are fixed in a:
1. 10% formal saline solution.
2. 20% formal saline solution.
3. 30% formal saline solution.
4. 40% formal saline solution.

179. The most important nutrient all animals need to survive is:
1. carbohydrates.
2. proteins.
3. water.
4. fat.

180. Which of the following barbiturates has the longest effect on patients?
1. Pentobarbital
2. Thiopental
3. Methohexital
4. Phenobarbital

181. Which of the following is a correct statement regarding the use of an alpha-2 adrenergic agonist on a horse during the postoperative period?
    1. It decreases the quality of recovery.
    2. It increases the number of attempts to stand.
    3. It slightly prolongs the recovery period.
    4. It doesn't affect the quality of recovery at all.

182. The immobilization of a joint or limb is an appropriate preoperative procedure for patients undergoing:
    1. orthopedic surgery.
    2. airway surgery.
    3. thoracic surgery.
    4. ophthalmological surgery.

183. Of the following, which piece of information is *least likely* to be included on a request form a technician would receive in the lab?
    1. A picture of the animal
    2. The owner's name and address
    3. A site diagram indicating where the sample was taken
    4. The name and address of the surgeon and his or her practice

184. Technicians often have to care for house pets other than cats and dogs. Among these pets are guinea pigs, hamsters, and rabbits. Which of the following statements is important for technicians caring for rabbits to keep in mind?
    1. Rabbits are always easy to anesthetize.
    2. Rabbits welcome new environments and people.
    3. Rabbits respond to the emotions of their caretakers.
    4. Rabbits benefit from newspaper lining in their cages.

185. Ultrasounds base their images of organs and tissues inside the animal on the time delay and amplitude of returning:
    1. shadows.
    2. lights.
    3. sounds.
    4. echoes.

186. Which of the following describes the general state of an animal in category IV of the American Society of Anesthesiologists Classification of Physical Status?
    1. A patient is apparently healthy and is undergoing an orchiectomy.
    2. A patient has a bone fracture but is not in shock or otherwise ill.
    3. A patient has a high fever and is severely malnourished.
    4. A patient suffers from extreme shock and severe dehydration.

187. A veterinary technician travels to a farm to treat an animal for *Anoplocephala perfoliata*, a common type of tapeworm. To remove the tapeworm, the technician administers an oral dose of pyrantel pamoate paste. The veterinary technician is *most likely* treating a:
    1. pig.
    2. horse.
    3. cow.
    4. chicken.

188. When should you count the swabs, needles, and sutures used during surgery?
    1. Before and after surgery
    2. Only during surgery
    3. Before and during surgery
    4. Only after surgery

189. A technician who is setting up for an incoming iguana should use a large aquarium or a large cat cage. The technician should line the aquarium or cage with:
    1. sand.
    2. gravel.
    3. alfalfa pellets.
    4. wood shavings.

190. All the following animals would be at risk of further injury during an MRI *except* a:
    1. dog with a bullet in its hind leg.
    2. cat that swallowed five paperclips.
    3. pregnant ferret with a broken leg.
    4. rabbit with eight skin staples on its back.

191. A technician treats a dog for spontaneous bleeding. The dog's owner tells the technician that the dog has experienced multiple bloody noses and has vomited blood twice in the past three days. The owner believes the dog may have ingested rat poison the family keeps in the garage. Which of the following forms of Vitamin K injections should the technician use as a treatment?

1. K2
2. K3
3. K4
4. K5

192. Before operating on a patient, you are supposed to take a blood sample to check the patient's BUN levels. You are *most likely* performing the test to check the patient's:

1. renal function.
2. respiratory function.
3. cardiac function.
4. muscular function.

193. Between operations, veterinary technicians often sterilize surgical equipment. Which of the following would technicians *least likely* sterilize using a chemical gas such as ethylene oxide?

1. Drills
2. Endoscopes
3. Drapes and gowns
4. Plastics and rubbers

194. When a cat's nasal passages are congested, it will *most likely*:

1. eat less.
2. sleep less
3. play less.
4. climb less.

195. A surgeon must perform a microvascular surgery on a ferret. Since the ferret has extremely small blood vessels, the instruments must be in excellent condition. All the following statements are true about general microvascular instruments *except*:

1. they should come in contact with other metal objects so that they stay magnetized.
2. they are often made of stainless steel or titanium with chromium tips.
3. they typically have a matte finish to prevent reflecting light into the surgeon's eyes.
4. they are designed to reduce the surgeon's chances of muscle fatigue and tremors.

196. A technician examines a dog that has fractured a tooth. The tooth has broken down to the pulp cavity and there's evidence of bleeding. It's obvious the patient is in pain as the pulp contains the tooth's sensory nerves and blood vessels. Which treatment will the technician *most likely* recommend for the dog's fractured tooth?

1. Ice it and wait for healing.
2. Apply a fluoride sealant.
3. Perform root canal therapy.
4. Remove the fractured tooth.

197. Which of the following combination of drugs is used to treat thunderstorm phobia and separation anxiety in dogs?

1. Atypical antipsychotics and tricyclic antidepressants
2. Anticonvulsants and monoamine oxidase inhibitors
3. Atypical antipsychotics and anticonvulsants
4. Tricyclic antidepressants and benzodiazepines

198. Which of the following threatens aseptic techniques and should be avoided in operating rooms?

1. Lighting fixtures that are flush with ceiling
2. Ventilation units
3. Waterproof, recessed electrical outlets
4. Forced-air heating units

199. Which of the following is an example of poor inventory-control techniques?

1. A veterinary technician reads the label of a medication to find out where to store it.
2. A veterinary technician checks and marks the inventory sheet while unloading supplies.
3. A veterinary technician makes notes about supplies that are running low.
4. A veterinary technician places new items in front of old items on storage shelves.

200. A correct statement concerning transporting patients with wounds involving penetrating foreign bodies is:
1. wounds should be dressed using cotton or wool gauze.
2. protruding foreign bodies should be cut close to the wound.
3. wounds should be cleaned using a general antiseptic ointment.
4. protruding foreign bodies should be removed before dressing the wound.

PRACTICE TEST 2: ANSWER KEY AND EXPLANATIONS

1. 2	41. 3	81. 2	121. 1	161. 3
2. 2	42. 2	82. 2	122. 3	162. 3
3. 1	43. 4	83. 1	123. 2	163. 2
4. 1	44. 1	84. 1	124. 3	164. 1
5. 1	45. 4	85. 4	125. 4	165. 1
6. 3	46. 1	86. 2	126. 2	166. 2
7. 2	47. 1	87. 1	127. 4	167. 2
8. 2	48. 2	88. 1	128. 4	168. 1
9. 4	49. 1	89. 4	129. 2	169. 2
10. 4	50. 4	90. 3	130. 1	170. 1
11. 2	51. 1	91. 3	131. 2	171. 2
12. 3	52. 3	92. 2	132. 2	172. 1
13. 3	53. 3	93. 4	133. 4	173. 3
14. 1	54. 4	94. 3	134. 4	174. 4
15. 1	55. 3	95. 1	135. 2	175. 3
16. 1	56. 3	96. 4	136. 3	176. 4
17. 4	57. 2	97. 4	137. 1	177. 3
18. 1	58. 1	98. 4	138. 1	178. 1
19. 4	59. 4	99. 1	139. 3	179. 3
20. 2	60. 3	100. 2	140. 1	180. 4
21. 3	61. 3	101. 2	141. 2	181. 3
22. 2	62. 2	102. 3	142. 3	182. 1
23. 4	63. 1	103. 1	143. 2	183. 1
24. 3	64. 2	104. 4	144. 3	184. 3
25. 2	65. 3	105. 4	145. 2	185. 4
26. 1	66. 1	106. 1	146. 1	186. 3
27. 2	67. 4	107. 2	147. 3	187. 2
28. 4	68. 3	108. 2	148. 2	188. 1
29. 2	69. 2	109. 3	149. 2	189. 3
30. 4	70. 2	110. 3	150. 2	190. 3
31. 2	71. 2	111. 4	151. 1	191. 1
32. 4	72. 2	112. 4	152. 4	192. 1
33. 3	73. 4	113. 2	153. 3	193. 3
34. 3	74. 2	114. 3	154. 1	194. 1
35. 1	75. 3	115. 3	155. 3	195. 1
36. 1	76. 4	116. 3	156. 2	196. 3
37. 4	77. 3	117. 4	157. 1	197. 4
38. 4	78. 3	118. 3	158. 1	198. 4
39. 3	79. 1	119. 3	159. 2	199. 4
40. 3	80. 3	120. 3	160. 2	200. 2

1. **The correct answer is 2.** Coronary vasoconstriction, among other factors, causes a decrease in cardiac output by 50% in most animals. Another factor is the baroreceptor reflex. Increased afterload, low catecholamine levels, and decreased myocardial oxygen consumption can all increase cardiac output, so choices 1, 3, and 4 incorrect.

2. **The correct answer is 2.** Often, geriatric patients take longer to recover than young patients. By scheduling geriatric patients before young patients, you give the geriatric patients more time during the day to recover, thereby reducing the likelihood of those patients having to spend another night at the hospital. Choice 1 is incorrect because geriatric, not young, patients are more likely to become stressed. Choices 3 and 4 are incorrect because geriatric patients have to eat and drink more often than young patients, which is another reason why geriatric patients should be scheduled for surgery before young patients.

3. **The correct answer is 1.** Premolars are primarily used for cutting, shearing, and holding. Incisors (choice 2) are used for cutting and nibbling. Molars (choice 3) are used for grinding. Canines (choice 4) are used for holding and tearing.

4. **The correct answer is 1.** As soon as a tissue sample is removed from an animal, the tissue immediately begins to die, and cell membranes begin to break down in a process called autolysis. Warm temperatures and high levels of humidity accelerate this process, so choice 2 is incorrect. Fixing tissues delays, rather than accelerates, deterioration of the cells, so choice 3 is incorrect. Tissues for standard histological examination should not be frozen for the test, so choice 4 is incorrect.

5. **The correct answer is 1.** Clients should not be skeptical of the veterinarian's treatments or instructions in a veterinarian-client-patient relationship. If the client refuses to follow or doubts the veterinarian's instructions, a veterinarian-client-patient relationship doesn't exist. Choices 2, 3, and 4 are all common traits of a successful veterinarian-client-patient relationship, so these choices are incorrect.

6. **The correct answer is 3.** A major disadvantage of performing fluoroscopic studies on animals is that the equipment used exposes veterinary personnel to a large amount of radiation. Technicians who know how to protect themselves properly from radiation should be among the only people who run these studies. Choice 1 is incorrect because the price of the test is worth the benefits of the test. Choice 2 is incorrect because being able to save images in different formats is a benefit of using fluoroscopic studies. Choice 4 is incorrect because fluoroscopic studies are quicker and easier to perform than angiographic catheterizations.

7. **The correct answer is 2.** The tape technique—which involves pressing a piece of clear adhesive tape to an area of the animal's skin, pulling it off, and inspecting the tape under a microscope—doesn't detect ringworm. Instead, hairs are removed and tested for ringworm infection. Choices 1, 3, and 4 are incorrect because the tape technique works for examining skin for bacteria, Malassezia, and surface mites.

8. **The correct answer is 2.** The equipment that is still sterile is the instrument that the technician opened without touching the paper to the instrument. Instruments are still sterile when they are open if they are opened correctly. Choice 1 is incorrect because instruments in wet packaging are not sterile. Choice 3 is incorrect because packages that have been punctured or otherwise opened improperly are not sterile. Choice 4 is incorrect because the technician's forearm touching the instrument made the instrument unsterile.

9. **The correct answer is 4.** Although smaller containers can be placed inside one large container, all containers (regardless of size or location) need detailed labels. Choices 1, 2, and 3 are incorrect because these statements are true. Toxicology specimens should never be washed; they should be submitted in leak-proof and sterile containers, and they should be collected fresh and delivered frozen.

10. **The correct answer is 4.** Many clinics don't line kennel floors with newspapers because newspapers don't warm patients. Newspapers are, however, readily available, easily disposable, and absorbent, so choices 1, 2, and 3 are incorrect.

11. **The correct answer is 2.** In dogs, amiodarone metabolizes to desethylamiodarone. Desethylamiodarone is often used to block fast-moving—not slow-moving—sodium channels, so choice 3 is incorrect. Amiodarone has a high iodine content and is structurally related to levothyroxine, making choices 1 and 4 incorrect.

12. **The correct answer is 3.** Atracurium doesn't cause sympathetic stimulation. Choices 1, 2, and 4 are incorrect because atracurium causes a release of histamine, doesn't affect intraocular pressure, and has indeterminate effects.

13. **The correct answer is 3.** Key-Gaskell Syndrome is rare, but when it does appear, it usually affects cats younger than 3 years, not older. Choices 1, 2, and 4 are incorrect as these statements are true regarding Key-Gaskell Syndrome. The syndrome is also known as feline dysautonomia, and it affects the autonomic nervous system. Research has shown more cases have been documented along the West Coast and Midwest regions of the United States than the East Coast.

14. **The correct answer is 1.** In a generally healthy patient, an anesthetic that is administered intravenously will most likely take effect within a few seconds. Intravenous drugs usually begin to work almost instantly. Choices 2, 3, and 4 are incorrect because intravenous drugs do not take a few minutes (choice 2), a few hours (choice 3), or a few days (choice 4) to take effect.

15. **The correct answer is 1.** One of the goals veterinary medical teams need to meet when anesthetizing a patient for ophthalmic surgery is to provide an immobile eye for the procedure. Choices 2, 3, and 4 are incorrect because the other goals teams have when anesthetizing a patient for this type of operation include providing a pain-free recovery, supporting cardiopulmonary function, and avoiding increases in intraocular pressure.

16. **The correct answer is 1.** Michel's trephine is most often used for bone biopsies. It cuts a circular hole in bones such as the skull, spine, or hip; is available in a range of diameters; and is manually operated. Therefore, choices 2, 3, and 4 are incorrect.

17. **The correct answer is 4.** Hydrochloric acid found in animal urine is typically used for the biochemical analyses of urea, ammonia, calcium, nitrogen, and uric acid. Choices 1 and 3 are incorrect because these substances are hazardous. Choice 2 is incorrect because acetic acid is used to determine levels of ascorbic acid.

18. **The correct answer is 1.** Praziquantel is used to treat the majority of tapeworm infections in companion animals such as dogs and cats. Praziquantel is not effective, however, in the treatment of *Spirometra mansonoides* and *Diphyllobothrium erinacei*. Niclosamide, buanamidine, and albendazole aren't so effective in the treatment of tapeworm infections in cats and dogs, so choices 2, 3, and 4 are incorrect.

19. **The correct answer is 4.** Dyspnea, or shortness of breath, is a life-threatening condition that should receive immediate medical care. Choices 1, 2, and 3 are incorrect because the condition is a true emergency. An example of a minor emergency is an insect sting, and an example of a serious emergency would be a bone or joint dislocation.

20. **The correct answer is 2.** During stage 2, patients have lost consciousness and move involuntarily. Stage 2 is when patients react to external stimulus with a struggling reflex. Choice 1 is incorrect because patients in stage 1 still have voluntary movement. Choices 3 and 4 are incorrect because patients have depressed reflexes during stages 3 and 4.

21. **The correct answer is 3.** Many times, technicians need to restrain the animal during feces collection so that the animal doesn't bite, scratch, or walk away during the collection. The best results come from fresh feces, rather than those samples picked up off the ground or collected from a litter box, so choice 1 is incorrect. Choice 2 is incorrect because urine should be collected first, not feces. A technician should never force feces from an animal as it may result in skin tissues in the sample or damage to the anal/rectal mucosa, so choice 4 is incorrect.

22. **The correct answer is 2.** Thiacetarsamide sodium is most frequently used to treat heartworms. Thiacetarsamide isn't recommended for the treatment of the types of worms in choices 1, 3, and 4, so those answers are incorrect.

23. **The correct answer is 4.** Rotary saws should not be used to perform surgery on animals. Choices 1, 2, and 3 are incorrect because oscillating saws, pneumatic drills, and electric drills are used in veterinary surgery.

24. **The correct answer is 3.** A dairy cow's serum and plasma may appear yellow during a colorimetric test because of the cow's high-carotene diet. Choices 1, 2, and 4 are incorrect because carotene is a chromatin that may change plasma and serum to yellow, not to red, green, or blue.

25. **The correct answer is 2.** When determining which intramuscular route to use while administering medication, a technician should avoid the gluteal muscles in the buttocks as well as the hamstring muscle group. Injections in these areas may cause bone or sciatic damage. Choices 1, 3, and 4 are incorrect because the areas in these options are all suitable injection sites.

26. **The correct answer is 1.** Although most normal, healthy patients have to fast for 12 hours before surgery, very young patients should not fast for long before anesthesia because they could become hypoglycemic. Choice 2 is incorrect because most healthy animals can have water, but not food, up to the time of the preoperative examination. Choice 3 is incorrect because patients undergoing abdominal surgeries generally fast longer than patients undergoing other surgeries. Choice 4 is incorrect because most patients must fast at least 12, not 4, hours before their surgeries.

27. **The correct answer is 2.** Rochester-Carmalt hemostatic forceps are designed so that the grooves of the instrument run longitudinally, making it easier to clamp down on stumps or pedicles. Choice 1 is incorrect because Halstead mosquito hemostatic forceps aren't large enough or strong enough to perform these tasks and are instead used on smaller point bleeders. Doyen intestinal forceps (choice 3) are tissue forceps used for stomach surgeries. Babock intestinal forceps (choice 4) are used only on connective tissues.

28. **The correct answer is 4.** Technicians should administer only nonirritant drugs via the subcutaneous route. Otherwise, the animal may experience irritation or necrosis of the skin. Choices 1, 2, and 3 are incorrect because the effects of subcutaneous injections are felt 30–45 minutes after injection, the area has a small supply of nerves, and the area has a large supply of blood vessels.

29. **The correct answer is 2.** X-rays are converted into visible light photons and photoelectrons in the image intensifier tube. X-rays originate in the fluoroscopic tube, which is located beneath the structure. The X-rays pass through the animal and into the image intensifier tube. From there, the photoelectrons go to the electrostatic lenses, which send the image to the output fluorescent screen. Choices 1, 3, and 4 are incorrect because these parts don't play a role in the conversion of X-rays to visible light photons.

30. **The correct answer is 4.** Morphine is an opioid that is often injected. Choices 1, 2, and 3 are incorrect because isoflurane, ether, and halothane are anesthetic drugs that are most often inhaled.

31. **The correct answer is 2.** Curettes are used for root planning and for the removal of subgigival calculus and soft tissue diseases in the periodontal pocket, so choice 3 is incorrect. Choice 1 is incorrect because curettes have one blade with two cutting edges. Choice 4 is not correct because a curette's cutting edges can be used on the front and the back of an animal's teeth.

32. **The correct answer is 4.** Surgeons would most likely not perform a dental prophylaxis, which includes tartar removal and the extraction of broken teeth, on a wild animal. Wild animals are generally not given routine patient treatments such as teeth cleanings. Scientists may perform abdominal surgeries (laparotomy), sterilization procedures, and flight restraint operations if necessary. Therefore choices 1, 2, and 3 are incorrect.

33. **The correct answer is 3.** In vitro, meaning "outside the body," hemolysis shouldn't occur if the plasma is successfully separated before transit. If a technician failed to separate the plasma, hemolysis may occur. Choices 1, 2, and 4 are incorrect because osmotic pressure, the size of the needle, and the vigorous shaking of samples can cause red cells to break and spill.

34. **The correct answer is 3.** The Robert Jones bandage technique requires the application of zinc oxide traction tape to the dorsal and ventral surfaces of

the foot. It decreases the chance the bandage will slip during application or during recovery. Choices 1, 2, and 4 are incorrect as the bandage can last only up to 2 weeks, the bandage doesn't necessarily have to cover the toes, and this technique requires a very large amount of cotton wool.

35. **The correct answer is 1.** The darkest parts of an exposed X-ray film indicate the presence of gas. Five gradients, from black to white, appear on exposed X-ray films according to the attenuation of tissues in the X-ray. While gas is the darkest opacity, mineral is the most opaque and appears as white on the film. Choices 2, 3, and 4 are incorrect because muscle appears as a gray color on X-ray films, while bone and mineral appear white. Fat appears as a dark gray or lighter black color on the films.

36. **The correct answer is 1.** Technicians administer anesthetics to horses intravenously through the jugular vein, which is located in the horse's neck. Choices 2, 3, and 4 are incorrect because cephalic, saphenous, and mesenteric veins aren't injected when anesthetizing a horse.

37. **The correct answer is 4.** Choices 1, 2, and 3 are incorrect because piperazine is recommended for use in dogs, cats, pigs, horses, and poultry with modular worm and pinworm infections. Technicians don't recommend its use in cattle. Praziquantel treats worms in cattle and sheep.

38. **The correct answer is 4.** Hypodermic injections are commonly administered via the subcutaneous, intramuscular, and intravenous routes, so choices 1, 2, and 3 are incorrect. They're not typically administered via epidural. Technicians decide which route is appropriate for each patient by assessing the patient's temperament, present condition, and how quickly the medication will cause a reaction.

39. **The correct answer is 3.** A bovine, or cow, has a dental formula of I0/6 C0/2 P6/6 M6/6, which equals 32 teeth. Each letter stands for a type of tooth: incisors (I), canines (C), premolars (P), and molars (M). In the formulas of adults, the letters are capitalized. Choices 1, 2, and 4 are incorrect because these formulas do not equal 32.

40. **The correct answer is 3.** If needle holders become too worn, they can very easily be replaced. Choice 1 is incorrect because they are one of the few instruments actually involved in metal-to-metal contact during surgeries. Choice 2 is incorrect because as they experience wear and tear, they grow sharp, not dull, and the risk of slicing necessary threads or materials increases. Large needles aren't recommended for placing delicate sutures because they don't offer so much control as the small needles, so choice 4 is incorrect.

41. **The correct answer is 3.** Generally, urine samples are collected and stored in plastic sample bottles. Choice 1 is incorrect because blood is collected in Vacutainers. Choice 2 is incorrect because cultures, not urine, are generally stored in Petri dishes. Choice 4 is not correct because glass vials are not generally large enough to collect and store urine samples.

42. **The correct answer is 2.** Occlusive dressings help to retain moisture within the wound. This moisture helps to eliminate necrotic tissue and allow for new, healthy tissue to form beneath the bandage. Choice 1 is incorrect because dry dressings absorb pus and other fluids. Choice 3 is incorrect because hemostatic dressings are used to control excessive bleeding. Choice 4 is incorrect because impregnated gauze dressings are applied to wounds that need to be kept moist from the outside, such as burns.

43. **The correct answer is 4.** When collecting cerebrospinal fluid, the area of the spine that technicians most frequently tap is the atlanto-occipital joint. They may also try the lumbosacral space. Although choices 1, 2, and 3 are areas of the spine, technicians don't typically tap them for CSF, so they are incorrect.

44. **The correct answer is 1.** A venous portography allows for further study of the portal venous system and requires an injection of positive contrast media into the animal's spleen or mesenteric vein, the vein responsible for draining blood from the small intestine. The mesenteric vein combines with the splenic vein to form the hepatic portal vein. Choices 2, 3, and 4 are incorrect because the cephalic, saphenous, and jugular veins don't

receive injections of positive contrast material during a venous portography.

45. **The correct answer is 4.** Of the methods listed, blood pressure monitoring is least likely to be used by technicians during a procedure, especially if they are performing the surgery in the field. In the clinic, they may have access to blood pressure monitoring and even electrocardiography tests, but many times technicians go without these monitoring methods while they work in the field. Choices 1, 2, and 3 are incorrect because these methods are used by veterinarians and technicians regardless of the procedure's location.

46. **The correct answer is 1.** Veterinarians may recommend the use of tofranil, elavil, or sinequan as an antidepressant. Choices 2 and 3 are incorrect because ativan and valium are benzodiazepines, and choice 4 is incorrect because risperdal is an atypical antipsychotic.

47. **The correct answer is 1.** If a person ingested chemical agents, he or she should seek medical attention as soon as possible. He or she should also try not to vomit. Choices 2, 3, and 4 are incorrect because they simply require flushing the contaminated area or dressing the wound. Unless irritation or bleeding persists, medical attention isn't necessary.

48. **The correct answer is 2.** When drawing blood from animals, a technician's first choice is always the jugular. If the jugular cannot be used for any reason, the technician will use the cephalic vein. Choices 1 and 4 are incorrect because these are not first-choice veins. Choice 3 is incorrect because the renal arteries are responsible for supplying the kidney with blood and should not be disturbed.

49. **The correct answer is 1.** Saffan has been proven to be most effective on cats. It's a steroid anesthetic, composed of alphaxalone and alphadolone. The typical dose for cats is 3–6 mg/kg. Choices 2, 3, and 4 are incorrect because this type of anesthetic at this particular amount is not used to anesthetize dogs, birds, or rabbits. When used in dogs, saffan causes a release of histamine.

50. **The correct answer is 4.** Technicians often have to perform emesis on a patient when the contents of the patient's stomach must be removed. Often times, this happens before surgery or before digestion is complete. Animals that swallow small toys or valuable items must be made to either vomit the item or wait until it moves into the bowel. Animals that have swallowed toxic materials are also made to vomit by emetics. Emesis is not recommended, however, when an animal has ingested a corrosive poison because bringing the poison back up through the stomach and throat will cause further harm and pain to the animal. Choices 1, 2, and 3 are incorrect as technicians can safely perform emesis in the situations presented in these options.

51. **The correct answer is 1.** An ideal operating room has one door to restrict or limit the flow of traffic into the operating room. The door should lead into the preparation room. Choices 2, 3, and 4 are incorrect because any more than one door would make for too much traffic in the operating room.

52. **The correct answer is 3.** Horses must fast for at least 12 hours before they receive anesthesia and surgery begins. They can drink water up to an hour before their surgery, but they cannot have any food during this time period. Choices 1 and 2 are incorrect because a horse should fast longer than 6 to 10 hours before surgery. Choice 4 is incorrect because a horse can fast for fewer than 14 hours.

53. **The correct answer is 3. Due to its caustic, or corrosive, characteristics, formaldehyde should not be used as an antiseptic or disinfectant. If the chemical is ever used, the handler should wear protective gloves. Choices 1, 2, and 4 are all chemical agents integrated in many common animal-safe antiseptics and disinfectants.**

54. **The correct answer is 4.** When the skin has been contaminated with a biological agent, one should never scrub the skin. Instead, one should rinse the area with water (choice 1), gently lather it with soap (choice 3), rinse again, and wipe with antiseptic cloths (choice 2).

55. **The correct answer is 3.** Although technicians may apply hot or cold cloths to a recumbent patient, they wouldn't place the patient in an ice bath. Technicians would, however, give the animal massages and apply pressure to the thorax to help drain secretions. This process is called coupage. They would also treat the patient with hydrotherapy. So, choices 1, 2, and 4 are incorrect.

56. **The correct answer is 3.** A right lateral decubital projection is achieved when an animal is lying on his or her right side. Positions are named after the points where the X-ray will enter the body and leave the body. Choice 1 is incorrect because ventrodorsal projection indicates the X-ray enters the ventral surface and exits the dorsal surface. Choice 2 is incorrect because in this position, the X-ray enters the cranium and exits the tail. Choice 4 is also incorrect as in this position the X-ray passes from the right side of the body to the left.

57. **The correct answer is 2.** The most common anesthetics veterinarians use on horses are standing sedations. These anesthetics allow horses to remain standing for both painful and difficult procedures. Choices 1, 3, and 4 are incorrect because these facts are true. Local anesthetics are used on horses to diagnose issues such as lameness, general anesthetics are used for procedures like cheek teeth removals, and the use of anesthetics in horses creates a higher level of safety for handlers, veterinarians, and the animal.

58. **The correct answer is 1.** When Beta-blockers are administered through an IV to dogs, veterinary technicians should monitor the animal's blood pressure and electrocardiograms. Large amounts of propranolol may have cardiac depressant effects. Technicians don't need to take X-rays (choice 2), monitor blood pressure and breathing sounds (choice 3), or watch bleeding or breath sounds (choice 4).

59. **The correct answer is 4.** Anyone entering the operating room should wash their hands with antiseptic scrubs for at least 2 full minutes. They should also have previously cut their nails short. Nails should be clean, without nail polish or false nails. Choices 1, 2, and 3 are incorrect because the times presented in these options are too short.

60. **The correct answer is 3.** A gray Vacutainer with a yellow collecting pot should contain a sample of whole blood and an anticoagulant of oxalate fluoride. Choice 1 is incorrect because heparin is found in green or green and orange Vacutainers with orange collecting pots. EDTA is found in lavender Vacutainers with pink collecting pots, so choice 2 is incorrect. Choice 4 is incorrect because sodium citrate anticoagulants are found in light blue Vacutainers.

61. **The correct answer is 3.** Although Bubble Wrap may be used to keep an animal warm, it's not often used to pad bandages. Instead, natural and man-made fibers such as foam, Soft Ban, and cotton wool are used as padding, so choices 1, 2, and 4 are incorrect.

62. **The correct answer is 2.** Morphine is an opioid. Choices 1 and 3 are incorrect because ketoprofen and aspirin are nonsteroidal anti-inflammatory drugs (NSAIDs). Choice 4 is incorrect because lidocaine is a local anesthetic.

63. **The correct answer is 1.** The first step a technician should complete when bandaging an animal's ear is to place a pad of cotton wool on the animal's head and fold the ear back onto the pad. The technician should then apply a dry dressing and place another pad of cotton wool over the ear. After applying a conforming bandage over the ear and under the chin, the technician may choose to anchor the bandage on the sides of the animal's head with the other ear. Finally, the technician should cover the bandage with adhesive tape. Choices 2, 3, and 4 are incorrect because these steps occur only after the ear is folded back onto a pad of cotton wool.

64. **The correct answer is 2.** A dog that is obese must be monitored closely during general anesthesia because obese patients can suffer many complications from anesthesia. Choices 1 and 3 are incorrect because those patients have normal heart rates, so they do not need to be monitored so closely as the obese dog. Choice 4 is incorrect because animals with normal weights are generally lower risk than animals with higher weights.

65. **The correct answer is 3.** Studies in 2006 indicated that use of acepromazine, an antipsychotic medication, did not lead to an increased risk of seizures when used to treat dogs. Veterinarians often recommend against the use of acepromazine for animals who are at risk of seizures, such as cats, squirrels, and bats, so choices 1, 2, and 4 are incorrect.

66. **The correct answer is 1.** Alcohols are drying agents, so choice 1 is correct. Because alcohols have a strong defatting effect, choice 2 is incorrect. Alcohols are more effective if they contain a small concentration of water, and they have a quick bacterial kill rate, so choices 3 and 4 are incorrect.

67. **The correct answer is 4.** Choices 1, 2, and 3 are incorrect because dentin, pulp cavity, and cementum are found in the teeth of both herbivores and carnivores. Only herbivores have infundibula, however, which are funnel-shaped indents at the tip of the tooth.

68. **The correct answer is 3.** The use of an autoclave is not necessary in this situation. It would be appropriate if cultures or used samples had contaminated a specific area, but when cleaning up a flammable liquid, the technician needs sand (choice 1), a bucket, water (choice 2), and detergent (choice 4). After absorbing the liquid, the sand can be shoveled into a bucket for disposal. The area of the spill can then be washed with soap and water.

69. **The correct answer is 2.** The veterinarian should complete the surgery because the animal is clearly suffering from the condition. But, the owner can no longer breed or show the dog because the dog's genetic condition has been changed. Choice 1 is incorrect because the animal is suffering and should be cared for. Choice 3 is incorrect because the veterinarian can treat the patient even if it is the first time she meets it and its owner. Choice 4 is incorrect because a veterinarian should not raise prices just because she is treating a show dog.

70. **The correct answer is 2.** A myelography allows technicians to examine an animal's spinal cord and help make a diagnosis of myelopathy, a condition in which the animal experiences clinical signs of pain, paralysis, or paresis. Choices 1, 3, and 4 are incorrect because these tests are not designed to allow further examination of the spinal cord. Celiographies allow for examination of the abdomen, angiographies allow for examination of the circulatory system, and epidurographies allow for further examination of the epidural space.

71. **The correct answer is 2.** Frequent visits by the owner are not advisable during an animal's recovery. Although a few visits while the animal is away from home is acceptable, technicians recommend against daily visits as it's often difficult for an animal to watch his or her owner walk away at the end of the visit. Choices 1, 3, and 4 are incorrect because giving the animal toys from home, frequently using the animal's name, and frequent grooming all aid in an animal's recovery as it keeps up morale and makes the patient feel special.

72. **The correct answer is 2.** Some veterinarians choose to use local anesthetics in combination with surgical anesthesia because the local technique doesn't affect cardiopulmonary function, which makes the combined technique useful for high-risk procedures. Choices 1, 3, and 4 are incorrect because these facts are true.

73. **The correct answer is 4.** Stomach tubes measuring 18 French are most appropriate for use with large dogs weighing more than 22.2 lbs. Choices 1, 2, and 3 would all be too small to use in this scenario.

74. **The correct answer is 2.** Fixed and centrally rotated eyeballs are a sign that the patient is in plane III. Other possible signs include increased abdominal respiration; dilated pupils; a fast, faint pulse; and decreased blood pressure. The other choices would suggest different planes.

75. **The correct answer is 3.** The second category measures the antiseptic's persistent microbial effectiveness. The first category measures the antiseptic's immediate efficacy, choice 1, meaning its effectiveness within the first 60 seconds after application. The third category measures the antiseptic's residual action, choice 4, or its effectiveness after five days of application. Choice 2 is incorrect because it's not one of the three categories.

76. **The correct answer is 4.** Since teeth are living structures that have their own nerve supply, blood vessels, and even lymph drainage, choices 1, 2, and 3 are incorrect. Domestic and wild animals experience tooth pain similar to humans. When teeth break or gums surrounding teeth are infected, the animal feels pain.

77. **The correct answer is 3.** Water turnover is the term used to describe the input and output of body water over a given period of time. Water shed, water monitoring, and water quality aren't veterinary or medical terms, so choices 1, 2, and 4 are incorrect.

78. **The correct answer is 3.** Colorimetry is the measurement of light that is absorbed or transmitted by a specific substance or solution at a particular wavelength. The light absorbed may be inverse or visual colorimetry while the light transmitted may

be direct or photometric colorimetry. Colorimetry is measured using a colorimeter. Choices 1, 2, and 4 are incorrect because colorimetry is not a measurement of color, sound, or waves.

79. **The correct answer is 1.** Technicians should feed animals in recovery food that is easy to digest, such as chicken or scrambled eggs. Food should be served warm; therefore, choice 2 is incorrect. If the animal doesn't eat the food within 15 minutes of being served, the technicians should take the food away. It's important not to leave the food out for a prolonged period of time, so choice 3 is incorrect. Technicians often place pieces of food on the paws or noses of their patients in an attempt to interest them in eating; they rarely place the food out of reach of a recovering animal that may be in pain. Therefore, choice 4 is incorrect.

80. **The correct answer is 3.** Upper gastrointestinal studies are designed to study the stomach and small intestine. They are typically recommended when an animal shows symptoms of small intestine disease such as vomiting, abdominal pain, or anorexia. If the bowel appears to be obstructed, a UGI is ordered to get a closer look at what may be obstructing the process. Choices 1, 2, and 4 are incorrect because UGIs don't examine the kidneys, liver, colon, or large intestine.

81. **The correct answer is 2.** One way to tell if a patient is unsuited for anesthesia is to take him or her on a walk. If the animal collapses or becomes distressed or dyspneic, a technician may conclude that placing the patient under anesthesia may threaten its life. Choices 1, 3, and 4 are incorrect because walking the animal—not examining its eating habits, observing its sleeping habits, or testing its urine or feces—is the best way to tell whether anesthesia is suitable.

82. **The correct answer is 2.** After the technician dropped the vial, she cleaned the mess and told her supervisor about the spill, so the worker acted responsibly and ethically. Choice 1 is incorrect because accidents can happen, and dropping a vial does not prove negligence. Choice 3 is not correct because the worker is not required legally or ethically to report the spill to the patient's owner. Choice 4 is not correct because veterinary

technicians (as well as veterinarians) can be reported for unethical behavior.

83. **The correct answer is 1.** Animals younger than 4 months old shouldn't fast more than 4 hours before the surgery. Larger or adult animals should fast up to 12 hours before the surgery. They can handle a longer fasting because their glycogen reserves are larger than those in newborns or young animals. Choices 2, 3, and 4 are incorrect because the times indicated are too long.

84. **The correct answer is 1.** In dogs, the first molar in the lower arcade and the fourth premolar in the upper arcade are larger than the rest and are referred to as carnassial teeth. The pairings in choices 2, 3, and 4 are incorrect because both teeth in these combinations aren't typically larger than the other teeth in a dog's mouth.

85. **The correct answer is 4.** Once you've finished using the microscope, you should turn down the rheostat, turn off the light, lower the stage, and finally clean the oil immersion lens, so choice 4 is correct. Once the lens is clean, you can cover the microscope and store it. Choices 1, 2, and 3 are incorrect because these steps occur before the action in choice 4.

86. **The correct answer is 2.** Newborn animals are poikilothermic, meaning their body temperature is easily influenced by their surroundings. Since newborns need to be warm, they are often placed in an incubator where the warm temperature is controlled and constant. The temperature of an incubator should be 86–91°F, or 30–33°C. Choice 1 is incorrect as the range is too low, and choices 3 and 4 are incorrect because the temperature ranges are too high.

87. **The correct answer is 1.** Granulation tissue is typically applied when the edges of the wound are separated, not close together. Choices 2, 3, and 4 are incorrect because these statements are true: the wound often becomes infected, scarring is often extensive, and healing can take place over weeks and even months.

88. **The correct answer is 1.** Rhinography studies are performed if an animal's nasal cavity may be obstructed, if there is pharyngeal discharge, or if there may be an upper airway obstruction.

Rhinography is a contrast study of the nasal cavity. Choices 2, 3, and 4 are incorrect because rhinography doesn't allow for further study of the cranial, pelvic, or thoracic cavities.

89. **The correct answer is 4.** When veterinarians administer ketamine to an animal, the animal's protective airway reflexes are maintained. Since the animal's eyes remain open, the pupil's dilate, and the cranial nerve reflexes become less depressed, choices 1, 2, and 3 are incorrect. Ketamine also causes the animal's heart rate to increase, breathing to reduce, and salivation to increase.

90. **The correct answer is 3.** Canine teeth may appear as tusks in some species of animals. They are located at the corners of the incisors and are typically pointed at the tip. Choice 1 is incorrect because premolars and molars are known as "cheek" teeth, not canines. Choices 2 and 4 are also incorrect because molars have flat, occlusal surfaces that animals use for grinding, and premolars in carnivores may have multiple, sharp points.

91. **The correct answer is 3.** Sevoflurane crosses the placental barrier very quickly and leads to fetal depression. Halothane (choice 1) is incorrect because it crosses the placental barrier, but does not result in fetal depression. Thiopental (choice 3) and etomidate (choice 4) are not correct because they cross the placental barrier, but have little to no effect on the fetus due to rapid clearance.

92. **The correct answer is 2.** Choice 2 is correct because the function of pulse oximeter is to chart the puppy's pulse rate and oxygen levels in the blood. Choice 1 is incorrect because an invasive blood pressure monitor tracks the direct systolic and diastolic blood pressures. Choice 3 is not correct because an ultrasonic Doppler unit can be used to chart pulse rate and rhythm. Choice 4 is incorrect because respiratory air movement can be monitored by a respiratory monitor.

93. **The correct answer is 4.** Of the group listed, bacterial endospores is the most resistant to disinfectants. Vegetative bacteria, choice 2, are typically the least resistant to disinfectants, followed by choice 3 and choice 1.

94. **The correct answer is 3.** Autonomic blocking drugs are often administered before anesthesia to prevent accidental stimulation of autonomic influences on visceral tissues. Many autonomic blocking drugs also act as antidotes to specific chemical toxins. Choices 1, 2, and 4 are incorrect because these types of blocking drugs (beta, neuromuscular, and acid) are not administered before anesthesia to prevent stimulation.

95. **The correct answer is 1.** Anisocoria is a condition in which the pupils of the eyes are different sizes. Choices 2, 3, and 4 are incorrect because cherry eye, entropion, and glaucoma are common eye/sight conditions in dogs, but each has different symptoms.

96. **The correct answer is 4.** Mucous membranes in cats and dogs should be pink, not white, and capillary refill time should be between 1 and 2 seconds. Dogs and cats may be healthy if their eyes are free of discharge, their ears are clean and odor-free, and they're able to move their limbs without any pain or resistance, so choices 1, 2, and 3 are incorrect.

97. **The correct answer is 4.** The loss of more than 20% of an animal's body weight puts the animal at risk of death during the procedure. If the animal survives the surgery, it will most likely experience a variety of postoperative complications. Choices 1, 2, and 3 are incorrect because the percentages are too low.

98. **The correct answer is 4.** An adult dog typically has 42 teeth. Puppies have 28 teeth, kittens have 26 teeth, and adult cats have 30. Therefore, choices 1, 2, and 3 are incorrect.

99. **The correct answer is 1.** The stage holds the slides on a compound microscope. Choice 2 is incorrect because the rotating turret is part of the nosepiece. Choice 3 is incorrect because the optical tube is within the body of the microscope. Finally, choice 4 is incorrect because the slides rest on the stage, which is above the substage condenser.

100. **The correct answer is 2.** An intravenous pyelogram (IVP) uses an X-ray and injectable dye to track the function of the kidneys, ureters, and urinary bladder. Choice 1 is incorrect because urohydropropulsion is a procedure used to help pass

bladder stones through the urethra. A CAT scan (computed tomography or CT scan) uses X-rays to scan the body for brain and spinal cord disorders, so choice 3 is incorrect. A perineal urethrostomy creates a new opening through which urine can pass and is performed on male cats with severe urinary blockages, so choice 4 is incorrect.

101. **The correct answer is 2.** A patient with a mild systemic disease would be placed in Class 2. Choice 1 is incorrect because Class 1 includes normal, healthy patients receiving elective procedures. Choice 3 is incorrect because Class 3 contains patients with severe systemic diseases that aren't incapacitating. Choice 4 is incorrect because Class 4 is for patients with severe systemic diseases that are a constant threat to the patients' lives. Class 5, the final categorization by the ASA, is for patients who aren't suspected to live past 24 hours, even if they receive treatment.

102. **The correct answer is 3.** The coccygeal artery is located on the ventral aspect of the base of the tail in cats and dogs. Choice 1 is incorrect because the femoral artery is located along the femur. Choice 2 is incorrect because the digital artery is on the carpus's palmar aspect. Finally, the lingual artery, choice 4, is located on the underside of the tongue and is only monitored in unconscious or anesthetized patients.

103. **The correct answer is 1.** Resorptive lesions are erosions of the tooth that primarily affect cats. Choices 2, 3, and 4 are incorrect because lizards, cattle, and horses are not affected by resorptive lesions.

104. **The correct answer is 4.** Chest compressions with high resonance are consistent with pneumothorax. Chest compressions with low resonance or even reduced breath sounds are consistent with lung consolidation, choice 3. Choices 1 and 2 are incorrect because these conditions are consistent with auscultation of rales and crepitus.

105. **The correct answer is 4.** The dog is experiencing a voracious, or increased, appetite. If the dog is losing, rather than gaining, weight after all the eating it is doing, it may have worms. As the owner didn't tell the vet that the dog was eating unnatural items, choice 1, pica, is incorrect. She also didn't say that the dog was eating its own feces, so choice

3, coprophagia, is incorrect as well. Finally, choice 2, polyuria, is incorrect because the dog hasn't shown any signs of increased urine production.

106. **The correct answer is 1.** Cats are solitary animals. When removed from their environment and placed in a busy area such as a veterinary clinic, they feel stressed and are more than willing to attack anything unfamiliar to them. Choices 2, 3, and 4 are incorrect as these animals are less likely than cats to attack.

107. **The correct answer is 2.** An MRI (magnetic resonance imaging) uses a magnetic field, radio waves, and a computer to produce images of the inside of the body. Choices 1 and 3 are incorrect because X-rays and CAT scans do not use a magnetic field to produce images of the body. Choice 4 is incorrect because a biopsy is the surgical removal of tissue, cells, fluids, or masses from the body.

108. **The correct answer is 2.** To test the corneal reflex, touch the surface of the patient's eye and wait for the patient to blink. This reflex is not present in the third stage of anesthesia. Choice 1 is incorrect because the palpebral reflex is tested by touching the corner of the eye. Choice 3 is incorrect because the pupillary reflex is tested with a light. Choice 4 is incorrect because a limb is pulled to test this reflex.

109. **The correct answer is 3.** Acyclovir is commonly used to treat Pacheco's disease in birds. It can also be used to treat feline herpes infections. The other drugs in choices 1, 2, and 4 (fluconazole, metronidazole, and oseltamivir) would not be used for this purpose.

110. **The correct answer is 3.** A decrease in blood flow and oxygen delivery is always the underlying cause of shock. Although tachycardia, circulatory collapse, and dehydration are associated with shock, they don't provoke the event; therefore, choices 1, 2, and 4 are incorrect.

111. **The correct answer is 4.** The dental formula—or the number of each type of tooth in the upper and lower arcade—for a grown cat is I6/6 C2/2 P6/4 M2/2. This means that the adult cat typically has 12 incisors, 4 canines, 10 premolars, and 4 molars. Choices 1 and 3 are incorrect because the lowercase

letters indicate that they are the dental formulas for baby animals. Choice 2 is incorrect because it's the dental formula for an adult pig.

112. **The correct answer is 4.** Ferrets have the ability to regurgitate. Rats, rabbits, and horses have a strong esophageal and stomach valve that prevents vomiting, so choices 1, 2, and 3 are incorrect.

113. **The correct answer is 2.** Once you've soaked the dirty glassware in disinfectant and then removed all debris, you should soak it in a fresh tub of detergent or an ultrasonic bath. After the bath, you would then rinse the glass in distilled water two to three times (choice 1). You'd drain the glassware (choice 3), and allow it to air dry or place it in a drying oven (choice 4).

114. **The correct answer is 3.** Feulgen stain is a type of staining method used to differentiate between chromosomal materials. Choice 1 is incorrect because Sudan 3 stain is used to differentiate between lipids. Choice 2 is incorrect because Van Gieson's stain is used to differentiate between different types of connective tissue. Choice 4 is incorrect because Gram's stain is used to differentiate between different types of bacteria.

115. **The correct answer is 3.** Cats become agitated if they don't receive privacy; therefore, placing them in an area where they cannot be seen by other animals will aid them in recovery. If a cage cannot be repositioned, putting a blanket over the cage may help. Choice 1 is incorrect because technicians should be sure to keep noise levels to a minimum as sudden, loud noises aggravate and frighten patients. Choice 2 is incorrect because even though speaking softly is recommended, making direct eye contact with a dog may be considered threatening. Choice 4 is incorrect as many animals, such as dogs, don't like to urinate or defecate in the area in which they are sleeping or spending time.

116. **The correct answer is 3.** The average gestation period for sheep is 147 days. Choices 1 and 2 are incorrect because the average gestation period is longer than 103 or 121 days. Choice 4 is incorrect because the average gestation period is shorter than 179 days.

117. **The correct answer is 4.** Optimum conditions for reading a radiograph include little to no glare around the periphery of the film. Choices 1, 2, and 3 are incorrect because optimum conditions also include a darkened room, bright lights, and dry films.

118. **The correct answer is 3.** The maximum weight of a surgical instrument pack being placed into an autoclave should be 5.5 kg. Loading heavier instrument packs may prevent proper steam penetration. Choices 1 and 2 are below the maximum weight. Choice 4 exceeds the maximum weight.

119. **The correct answer is 3.** The enamel is the outermost layer of an animal's tooth. It covers the crown of the tooth and is the hardest tissue in the entire body. Choice 1 is incorrect because the apex is the root of the tooth. Choices 2 and 4 are incorrect because the dentin is just beneath the enamel but surrounds the pulp, which is the innermost layer of the tooth.

120. **The correct answer is 3.** Universal sterile containers, which are generally used to collect urine and fecal samples, are made of either plastic or glass. They typically hold about 30 ml of fluid, not 300 ml, so choice 4 is incorrect. They are also small, wide-mouthed bottles, not large, narrow-mouthed bottles, so choices 1 and 2 are incorrect.

121. **The correct answer is 1.** Nephritis, or inflammation of the kidney, is a condition in which polydipsia, or increased thirst, is a symptom. A common side effect of cystic calculi, prostatic enlargement, and obstruction of the urinary tract is dysuria, or painful or difficult urination. Choices 2, 3, and 4 are incorrect because polydipsia is not a symptom of these conditions.

122. **The correct answer is 3.** Norepinephrine activates α-vascular receptors and causes vasoconstriction, which means that peripheral resistance increases and renal and femoral blood flows decrease. Choices 1, 2, and 4 are incorrect because these combinations of effects do not occur during vasoconstriction.

123. **The correct answer is 2.** Isoproterenol is a myocardial stimulant that increases the strength of myocardial contractile forces and accelerates

heart rate. Choice 1 is incorrect because it is independent of, rather than dependent on, changes in venous returns. Choice 3 is incorrect because it is 10–20, not 30–40, times more active in the heart than epinephrine. Choice 4 is incorrect because isoproterenol causes an increase in the rate of pressure changes in the ventricular chambers rather than a decrease.

124. **The correct answer is 3.** An ideal operating room would have a temperature of 70°F and a humidity level of approximately 50%. Choices 1 and 4 are incorrect because the temperatures are too cool, and choice 2 is incorrect because the humidity level is too high.

125. **The correct answer is 4.** An ideal antiseptic should cause little skin irritation or interference. It also has a low toxicity level, not a high toxicity level as indicated in choice 1. Choice 2 is incorrect because it should have high penetrability, not low penetrability. Choice 3 is incorrect because it should perform a broad spectrum of activities, rather than a narrow one.

126. **The correct answer is 2.** Although many people incorrectly identify this process as cold sterilization, choice 1, the correct name is immersion disinfection. The disinfectant the dog's owner chooses to use should be EPA-registered and will kill most of the infected organisms left on the items. Choices 3 and 4 are incorrect because these processes don't involve soaking small objects in disinfectant.

127. **The correct answer is 4.** Choices 1, 2, and 3 are incorrect because before a veterinarian examines the animal's respiratory rate, breath sounds, or depth of breathing, he or she will observe the animal's attitude, walk, and nutritional status.

128. **The correct answer is 4.** When using the coarse focus, you should adjust the focus knobs slowly to find the right focus. The coarse focus is more sensitive, so going slowly ensures that you will more easily find the correct focus. Choices 1, 2, and 3 are incorrect because those are true statements about microscopes.

129. **The correct answer is 2.** Cyclic vomiting is defined as reoccurring instances of vomiting. This type of vomiting occurs in four stages: symptom-free interval phase, prodrome phase, vomiting phase, and recovery phase. Bilious vomiting is vomiting of bile, while stercoraceous vomiting is the vomiting of feces. Since the cat's vomit shows no signs of bile or feces, choices 1 and 4 are incorrect. Choice 3 is incorrect as the technicians didn't indicate the cat was forcefully vomiting without first retching.

130. **The correct answer is 1.** A positive contrast cystography, or a cystogram, would be the most appropriate test to perform when evaluating bladder position and bladder wall integrity. Choices 2 and 4 are incorrect because negative contrast cystography, also known as pneumocystography, is least preferred because of a high risk of air embolism. Choice 3 is incorrect because double contrast cystographies are most helpful when assessing calculi or mural masses.

131. **The correct answer is 2.** Many veterinarians recommend pharmacological intervention in addition to behavior modification therapies to decrease compulsivity in domestic animals. This combination may also be used to decrease arousal and excitability and increase or promote behavioral calming, which makes choices 1, 3, and 4 incorrect.

132. **The correct answer is 2.** The liver metabolizes anesthetic drugs and produces both plasma proteins and coagulation factors. Animals with liver disease may experience blood thinning and longer effects of anesthetics. Choices 1, 3, and 4 are incorrect because the lungs, heart, and kidneys have different responsibilities.

133. **The correct answer is 4.** The presence of blood in an animal's urine is called hematuria. Choice 1 is incorrect as anuria occurs when an animal is unable to pass urine. Choice 2 is incorrect because dysuria is painful or difficult urination. Choice 3, oliguria, is the passing of a decreased amount of urine.

134. **The correct answer is 4.** Phenothiazines, or sedatives, increase the risk of extrapyramidal symptoms such as rigidity, tremor, or akinesia. Choices 1 and 3 are incorrect because the ability to achieve arousal and coordinated motor skills are not typically affected by phenothiazine. This agent decreases spontaneous motor activity in animals, however, which makes choice 2 incorrect.

135. **The correct answer is 2.** The pelvic limb swing stops animals from bearing weight on their hind legs and allows animals to move their joints. This immobilizer is used most often to help bone fractures and joint damage heal. Choice 1 is incorrect because the immobilizers described in this choice are hobbles. Choices 3 and 4 are not correct because they describe a leg cast (choice 3) and a carpal flexion bandage (choice 4).

136. **The correct answer is 3.** Tubular bandages are frequently used to wrap tails and limbs. They are made of elasticized cotton or nylon and are applied using an applicator. Choice 4 is incorrect because crepe bandages are generally used on larger body areas such as the head and abdomen. Choice 1 is incorrect as these bandages are large, but don't have the ability to conform to a specific area. Choice 2 is not correct because cohesive bandages are not generally used to bandage tails.

137. **The correct answer is 1.** Samantha is acting unethically as she is listing her membership in an organization of which she is no longer a member. Choice 2 is incorrect because technicians should work hard to continue their educations. Choice 3 is incorrect because it is ethical to share patient information when the public health is at risk. Choice 4 is incorrect because it is ethical for technicians to collaborate to ensure the best possible care for their patients.

138. **The correct answer is 1.** Catheterization is performed easily in male dogs and cats, but female cats rarely receive catheterization. If a catheter is required, female cats are sedated. Choices 2, 3, and 4 are incorrect because it's more common for male dogs, female pigs, and male horses to receive catheterization than female cats.

139. **The correct answer is 3.** Polydioxanone is the suture material that takes the longest to absorb at 180 to 120 days. Choice 1 is incorrect because polyglactin 910 takes 56 to 70 days to absorb. Choice 2 is incorrect because polyglycolic acid takes 60 to 90 days to absorb. Choice 4 is incorrect because poliglecaprone 25 takes 90 to 120 days to absorb.

140. **The correct answer is 1.** The arm of the microscope connects the base with the stage. The rheostat (choice 2) for the light source adjusts the level of light. The illuminator (choice 3) is located on the base and is the microscope's light source. The condenser (choice 4) is located above the light source, and it condenses the light into a small beam.

141. **The correct answer is 2.** Veterinary technicians prefer to take an animal's temperature via its rectum. This process should take 1 to 2 minutes. If a technician cannot use this method, he or she should use the axilla (the area beneath the arm where the arm meets the shoulder) or the external ear canal. Choices 1, 3, and 4 are incorrect as these parts are acceptable, but not preferable, areas in which to take an animal's temperature.

142. **The correct answer is 3.** Pyrexia, or increased body temperature, can be caused by infections, convulsions, and excitement, so choices 1, 2, and 4 are incorrect. Hypothermia is the word for decreased body temperature, so choice 3 is correct.

143. **The correct answer is 2.** Many behavioral drugs are made of water-soluble salts such as fluoxetine and buspirone because these salts allow for rapid dissolution in the gastrointestinal tract and good permeability in the intestine. Choices 1 and 4 are incorrect because these drugs allow for rapid, not slow, dissolution. Choice 3 is incorrect because they allow for good, not poor, permeability in the intestine.

144. **The correct answer is 3.** The horse has a complicated fracture, meaning the broken bone fragments have damaged the area surrounding the bone. Choices 1, 2, and 4 are incorrect because these fractures don't result in additional damage to the surrounding areas. An incomplete fracture occurs when the bone breaks on one side, but doesn't split into two pieces. A simple fracture occurs when the bone breaks cleanly into two separate pieces. Had the horse broken his leg in two separate, distanced places, it would have sustained a multiple fracture.

145. **The correct answer is 2.** Ultrasounds have eliminated the need for many radiographic exams similar to venous portography, celiography, and esophagography. Ultrasounds allow veterinarians to inspect the same organs as these exams, but in a more efficient and safer ways. Although ultrasounds are quite popular, they cannot do the

work of X-rays, computed tomographies (CTs), or MRIs; therefore, choices 1, 3, and 4 are incorrect.

146. **The correct answer is 1.** One common side effect of general anesthesia is low body temperature, so choice 1 is correct. Choices 2, 3, and 4 are incorrect because reduced body weight, infection, and hemorrhaging are not common side effects of general anesthesia.

147. **The correct answer is 3.** Aminoglycosides are thermodynamically stable within a vast range of pH values and temperatures. They also have excellent solubility in water, poor lipid solubility, and molecular weights of 400–500 g/mol, making choices 1, 2, and 4 incorrect.

148. **The correct answer is 2.** If technicians don't plan on using serum or plasma samples immediately, they should clearly label the samples and place them in a freezer at –4°F, or –20°C. Choice 1 is incorrect because the temperature is too cold, and choices 3 and 4 are incorrect because the temperatures are too warm to store serum or plasma samples.

149. **The correct answer is 2.** Crypotorchidism is a procedure that involves the extraction of a testicle. Some horses are born before their testicles drop. This condition is called testicular retention. The severity of the retention, or where the testicle is located, predicts the type of cryptorchidism a surgeon must perform. Choices 1, 3, and 4 are incorrect because cryptorchidism doesn't involve the amputation of limbs, the removal of tumors, or the resetting of bones.

150. **The correct answer is 2.** A technician would cut a rabbit's molars, or cheek teeth, with molar cutters and smooth the ridges with a diamond burr. Choices 1 and 4 are incorrect because molar luxators and extraction forceps are used to remove, not trim, teeth. Choice 3 is incorrect because even though a soft tissue protector is part of a diamond burr, the technician also needs molar cutters to perform the task.

151. **The correct answer is 1.** Sufficient skin scrapings occur only when petechial bleeding has been achieved. This involves scraping off the top layer of skin only. Choice 2 is incorrect because a skin scraping down the hypodermis layer is unnecessary and painful. Choice 3 is incorrect because if the sample is not immediately tested, it's placed in a container, scalpel and all. The technician should squeeze the skin and push the bacteria and parasites toward the surface of the skin to obtain a sample. Choice 4 is incorrect because the bacteria need a push toward the surface.

152. **The correct answer is 4.** If visiting the patient is necessary, consulting veterinarians examine the patient in the presence of the attending veterinarian. Although the consulting veterinarian may perform the assessment or recommend treatment, the attending veterinarian is still in charge of the veterinarian-client-patient relationship, so choice 3 is incorrect. Choice 1 is incorrect because consulting veterinarians sometimes don't charge for their services at all. This differs from attending veterinarians, who almost always charge fees. Consulting veterinarians typically offer their expert opinions on lab results, test results, and diagnostic images. They rarely visit with the patient; therefore, they don't perform many physical exams or patient observations, making choice 2 incorrect.

153. **The correct answer is 3.** Technicians can provide copies of records to clients without a court order. If the records are requested, the technician must fill out a written release to document the request. Choices 1, 2, and 4 are incorrect because these statements are true. The information in medical records should comply with state and federal standards, the information is confidential, and the records are considered the property of the practice or clinic in which they were composed.

154. **The correct answer is 1.** A computerized, mathematical cross-sectioned image of a cat's brain can be obtained with a CT, or computed tomography. CTs send X-ray transmissions through slices of thin patient tissue to create images. Choices 2, 3, and 4 are incorrect because each of these processes assess different areas and don't result in computerized, cross-sectional images.

155. **The correct answer is 3.** Epinephrine can be given to patients with anesthetic to make the anesthetic work for more time by decreasing blood flow. As the blood flow slows, the anesthetic moves more slowly around the body, so it works longer. Choices 1 and 2 are incorrect because epinephrine does not increase blood flow. Choice 4 is incorrect because

epinephrine makes the anesthetic work for more, not less, time.

156. **The correct answer is 2.** Approximately 15–30 ml/kg of an animal's total body water is eliminated due to insensible losses, such as evaporation, every day. Small animals or immature animals are at a greater risk of insensible losses than larger, adult animals. Choice 1 is incorrect because the amount is too low and choices 3 and 4 are incorrect because the amounts are too high.

157. **The correct answer is 1.** One of the many names for a procedure involving an incision into the abdomen is *celiotomy*. Choice 2 is incorrect because this procedure involves the brain. Choice 3 is incorrect because cystotomy is a type of bladder surgery. Choice 4 is incorrect because this procedure involves kidney removal.

158. **The correct answer is 1.** Although not common, some species of lizards do grow teeth on their palates. Typically, though, lizards have sharp, tricuspid teeth that grow on their maxilla, dentary, and premaxilla bones. Choices 2, 3, and 4 are incorrect because technicians would expect to find teeth growing in these locations.

159. **The correct answer is 2.** Formalin, which consists of 40% formaldehyde, is used in many laboratories to preserve valuable tissue samples by hardening, or fixing, them. Although choices 1, 3, and 4 are antiseptics or disinfectants, they don't have the abilities that formalin does. Glutaraldehyde is effective in fighting a wide range of bacterial activity, but it doesn't preserve tissue. Bleach is cheap and effective in eliminating fungi, spores, and viruses, but it also doesn't fix tissue samples. Triclosan isn't toxic, nor is it harsh on skin, but it also isn't used in preserving tissue samples.

160. **The correct answer is 2.** After surgery, it's important to take care when bandaging a patient's head. Anesthesia can effect the respiration of a patient, so special care should be taken around the head, throat, and abdomen so no breathing complications arise. Since joints (choice 1), legs (choice 3), and paws (choice 4) have nothing to do with respiration, these choices are incorrect.

161. **The correct answer is 3.** Scientists have proven that using buspirone in felines regulates the state of high arousal and decreases the occurrence of feline urine spraying by 55%. Buspirone doesn't affect cats' memory or psychomotor skills, nor does it induce a panic-like state, so choices 2 and 4 are incorrect. Effects of buspirone are evident after several weeks of administrating the drug, so choice 1 is also incorrect.

162. **The correct answer is 3.** Aseptic techniques are techniques used to keep an operating room sterile. When people talk, their breath releases bacteria into the air. Therefore, keeping talking to a minimum will help keep the room sterile. Choices 1, 2, and 4 are incorrect because aseptic techniques have nothing to do with keeping the patient happy (choice 1), maintaining surgeons' concentration (choice 2), or keeping the attention of the surgical team (choice 4).

163. **The correct answer is 2.** If a pet experiences an extreme buildup of plaque or tartar, this could lead to swollen and sore gums, a loss of teeth, and even infections in the liver, heart, kidneys, and lungs. Choices 1, 3, and 4 are incorrect answers because these events can easily occur if an animal's mouth continues to grow bacteria. Choice 2 is the correct answer because a buildup of tartar will not lead to duplicate canine teeth. The development of duplicate canine teeth is a common genetic defect in cats, but it is inherited and not caused by plaque and tartar.

164. **The correct answer is 1.** Cats should be housed in areas that are at least 50°F, or 10°C, at all times. Environments in which dogs spend their sleeping hours should also never drop below 50°F. Choices 2, 3, and 4 are incorrect because these temperatures are too high.

165. **The correct answer is 1.** Patients that are very young and patients undergoing cardiovascular surgery sometimes receive hypothermia as a form of anesthesia, so choice 1 is correct. Choices 2, 3, and 4 are incorrect because patients undergoing dental, ophthalmological, and joint surgeries do not usually receive hypothermia as a form of anesthesia.

166. **The correct answer is 2.** Fluoxetine is used to treat dominance-related aggression, inter-dog aggression, and acral lick dermatitis in dogs. It is also recommended for compulsive disorders and

canine separation anxiety. In humans, fluoxetine is used to treat obsessive-compulsive disorders, eating disorders, and generalized anxiety. Choice 1, dapoxetine, is not used to treat these behaviors in dogs, and choices 3 and 4 are incorrect because these SSRIs (zimelidine and indalpine) have been discontinued for many years.

167. **The correct answer is 2.** When you are preparing for surgery, your first step should be to change into a scrub suit. After you put on the suit, you can put on a cap and mask (choice 1), scrub for surgery (choice 3), put a sterile gown, and put on sterile gloves (choice 4).

168. **The correct answer is 1.** To avoid self-exposure to harmful toxins when anesthetizing animals, veterinary technicians should empty the rebreathing bags using the scavenging systems by opening the pressure release valve completely, not by detaching the bag from the cylinder. Emptying the bags this way may expose the technician to toxins. Choices 2, 3, and 4 are incorrect because these methods ensure the safety of veterinarians and technicians. To keep the environment safe for all, vaporizers should be placed outside of the operating area, the circuits should be examined for leaks regularly, and scavenging systems should be used.

169. **The correct answer is 2.** During dental polishing, you should keep the prophy cup moving at all times in order to avoid heating the tooth. This is the only key reason to keep the prophy cup moving, as overheating the tooth can cause damage. Choices 1, 3, and 4 are incorrect because constantly moving the cup will not help reach more of the tooth, remove more plaque, or minimize the required pressure.

170. **The correct answer is 1.** Synovial fluid, which is located in joints, is collected through a process called athrocentesis. This can be performed on an anesthetized or a conscious animal. Choice 2 is incorrect because thoracocentesis is the extraction of thoracic fluid, and choice 3 is incorrect because abdominocentesis involves extracting fluid from the abdominal cavity. Finally, pericardiocentesis is the process used to remove fluid from around the heart, so choice 4 is also incorrect.

171. **The correct answer is 2.** One way a technician can make a dog feel comfortable before restraining or handling him is to crouch down in front of him

so the technician is at eye level with the animal. Choice 1 is incorrect, as direct eye contact with a frightened dog may appear threatening. Choice 3 is also incorrect because sitting on the ground in front of the dog makes the technician vulnerable. Choice 4 is incorrect because a technician who is restraining a dog should talk to the animal in calm, soothing tones, not high-pitched or excited tones.

172. **The correct answer is 1.** Anuria, or the inability to pass urine, is a result of shock. Anuria may also be caused by FUS, obstruction of the urinary tract, infection, or renal failure. Choices 2, 3, and 4 are incorrect because there's no indication that shock may cause painful or difficult urination, increased urine production, or increased thirst in animals.

173. **The correct answer is 3.** Brachycephalic dogs are most likely to have airway blockages while they are under anesthesia because of the abnormal structure of their respiratory systems. Hypothermia (choice 1), cardiomyopathy (choice 2), and spinal instability (choice 4) are not related to the respiratory system, so they are not common complications of brachycephalic dogs.

174. **The correct answer is 4.** Splints are not a way to reduce dead space around wounds. Splints hold broken or injured body parts in place to help them heal, but they do not generally help reduce dead space around wounds. Compression bandages, drainage, and Robert Jones bandages, however, help eliminate dead space and help wounds heal. Therefore, choices 1, 2, and 3 are incorrect.

175. **The correct answer is 3.** Abdominocentesis is designed to detect an increase in the volume of peritoneal fluid in the abdomen. Synovial fluid is collected through a process called athrocentesis and is located within joints. Thoracocentesis is the extraction of thoracic fluid and cerebrospinal fluid is found in the spine, not the abdomen. Choices 1, 2, and 4 are incorrect.

176. **The correct answer is 4.** Stainless steel cages are very expensive to purchase. Depending on the size of the clinic, buying multiple cages could cost hundreds of dollars. Since these cages are easy to clean, are safe for many types of animals, and are indestructible, they might be worth the price. Alternative accommodations include brick kennels with tile floors and wooden kennels, but both may

present various dangers to animals. Choices 1, 2, and 3 are incorrect because these facts are true.

177. **The correct answer is 3.** Ketoprofen is a nonsteroidal anti-inflammatory drug that is often used as an analgesia following surgery. Morphine, fentanyl, and butorphanol are opioids—not NSAIDs—so choices 1, 2, and 4 are incorrect.

178. **The correct answer is 1.** After a technician performs a biopsy slated for histopathology, he or she will place the tissue sample in a solution composed of 10% formal saline. This solution is created by diluting formalin in a saline solution. Choices 2, 3, and 4 are incorrect because the percentage of formalin in the solutions is too high.

179. **The correct answer is 3.** The only time an animal should be denied water is if he or she is consistently vomiting. Otherwise, quality drinking water should be available to all animals at all times. While many animals can survive the loss of at least half their body fat or proteins, they cannot survive without water. Any more than a 15% loss of body water can cause the death of an animal. Choices 1, 2, and 4 are incorrect because animals can survive on a loss of carbohydrates, proteins, and fats.

180. **The correct answer is 4.** Phenobarbital is a long-lasting barbiturate that is used in anesthesia. Pentobarbital (choice 1), thiopental (choice 2), and methohexital (choice 3) are all short-term barbiturates used as anesthesia, so those choices are incorrect.

181. **The correct answer is 3.** The use of alpha-2 adrenergic agonists on horses during the postoperative period slightly prolongs the recovery period. It also increases the quality of recovery and decreases the number of attempts the horse must make to stand after the operation, so choices 1 and 2 are incorrect. The horse is affected by this agonist; therefore, choice 4 is also incorrect.

182. **The correct answer is 1.** Orthopedic surgery could require you to immobilize a joint or a limb. Choices 2, 3, and 4 are incorrect because airway surgery, thoracic surgery (surgery on the chest), and ophthalmological surgery (surgery on the eye) do not affect the joints and limbs, and they do not require limb immobilization.

183. **The correct answer is 1.** Request forms don't come attached with pictures of the animals from which the samples were taken. Other information identifying the animal will be included on the form, however. These details include the animal's name, species, age, sex, and the animal's clinical history. Choices 2, 3, and 4 are incorrect because this information is typically included on every request form.

184. **The correct answer is 3.** Rabbits may respond to the emotions, moods, or attitudes of their caretakers. It's important that any technician caring for rabbits remains calm. Rabbits respond to stress, and if a technician caring for a rabbit is stressed, the rabbit will become stressed. This trait makes choices 1 and 2 incorrect, as rabbits can easily become stressed in new environments, making it difficult to anesthetize them. Choice 4 is also incorrect as newspaper lining can cause sore hocks and stain rabbit coats.

185. **The correct answer is 4.** Ultrasounds send sound waves into the body of the animal and form images based on the echoes of sound energy that bounce off the tissues and organs. Although ultrasounds receive 99% of their information in the form of echoes, approximately 1% of the time they receive information from actual sound. This is not often enough to make choice 3 correct, however. Choices 1 and 2 are incorrect because ultrasounds don't detect shadows or lights.

186. **The correct answer is 3.** A patient that has a high fever and is severely malnourished would fit in category IV of the American Society of Anesthesiologists Classification of Physical Status. Category IV patients are patients that have life-threatening health problems and have a chance of surviving with medical attention. Choices 1, 2, and 4 are incorrect because they describe patients in category I (choice 1), category II (choice 2), and category V (choice 4) of the American Society of Anesthesiologists Classification of Physical Status.

187. **The correct answer is 2.** The technician in this scenario is most likely treating a horse. *Anoplocephala perfoliata* is a tapeworm most commonly found in horses, not pigs, cows, or poultry; therefore, choices 1, 3, and 4 are incorrect. The most effective way to treat this condition in

horses is to administer pyrantel pamoate paste orally.

188. **The correct answer is 1.** You should count surgery tools such as swabs, needles, and sutures before and after surgery. Counting these instruments before surgery tells you the exact number of each instrument. Counting the instruments after surgery helps you make sure no instruments were left inside the patient during surgery. Choices 2 and 3 are not correct because you don't need to count the instruments during surgery. Choice 4 is incorrect because you need to count the instruments before surgery, too.

189. **The correct answer is 3.** The most appropriate and comfortable bedding for an iguana is alfalfa pellets. This bedding is not only suitable because it is comfortable for sleeping, but it is also suitable because iguanas consume the pellets. Choices 1, 2, and 4 are incorrect because sand, gravel, and wood shavings can injure an iguana. These materials may lead to impaction or even gastric obstruction.

190. **The correct answer is 3.** The only animal that wouldn't be at risk during an MRI is the pregnant ferret suffering from a broken leg. MRIs are magnetic; therefore, it's highly recommended that any patients with some sort of metal within their body are not placed within an MRI. Choices 1, 2, and 4 are incorrect because bullets, paperclips, and staples are magnetic and may be pulled out of the animal's body when the technician turns on the machine.

191. **The correct answer is 1.** Rat poisons contain chemicals that act as anticoagulants, which alter the performance of Vitamin K. Vitamin K is responsible for blood clotting. K2, or menaquinone, has the ability to block the blood-thinning effects of many anticoagulants. Choices 2, 3, and 4 are used for issues other than thickening blood. For example, Vitamin K_3 may produce anticancer effects in humans and some animals.

192. **The correct answer is 1.** Testing a patient's blood urea nitrogen (BUN) is usually used to check the patient's renal function. If the patient has a high BUN level, it could indicate problems with the renal system. Choices 2, 3, and 4 are incorrect because

urea (the protein that is tested) is not an indicator of respiratory, cardiac, or muscular functions.

193. **The correct answer is 3.** Technicians use an autoclave to sterilize drapes and gowns, not ethylene oxide. To sterilize drills, endoscopes, and plastic and rubber instruments, however, technicians expose these instruments to ethylene oxide for approximately 12 hours and then ventilate the items for another 24 hours. Choices 1, 2, and 4 are incorrect because technicians commonly use a chemical gas such as ethylene oxide to sterilize these instruments.

194. **The correct answer is 1.** Since the ability to smell is closely linked to the ability to taste, cats will most likely eat less when their nasal passages are congested. The congestion affects their olfactory function and minimizes their ability to taste what they're eating. Choices 2, 3, and 4 are incorrect because a congested nasal passage will affect a cat's willingness to eat more than its willingness to sleep, play, or climb.

195. **The correct answer is 1.** Microvascular instruments are made of stainless steel or titanium to decrease the chances of magnetization. Surgeons don't want their instruments magnetized, so they attempt to keep them away from other metal objects whenever possible. Choices 2, 3, and 4 are incorrect answers because they are all characteristics of microvascular instruments.

196. **The correct answer is 3.** The technician will most likely recommend root canal therapy to treat the dog's fractured tooth. Typically, technicians and veterinarians avoid recommending tooth extraction as it takes weeks for the wound to heal properly and the dog is left without tooth function, so choice 4 is incorrect. Since the fracture exposed the tooth's pulp cavity, applying fluoride sealant (choice 2) or ice (choice 1) would not be preferred treatments.

197. **The correct answer is 4.** Veterinarians use a combination of tricyclic antidepressants and benzodiazepines to treat such behavioral conditions as thunderstorm phobia and separation anxiety in dogs. Choices 1, 2, and 3 are incorrect because these combinations of drugs aren't used to treat these issues in dogs.

198. **The correct answer is 4.** Forced-air heating units threaten aseptic techniques and should not

be installed in operating rooms. The air from the heating unit can carry dust and microbes that can contaminate the operating room. Choices 1, 2, and 3 are incorrect because these elements help maintain aseptic techniques in operating rooms.

199. **The correct answer is 4.** A veterinary technician placing new items in front of old items on storage shelves is an example of poor inventory-control techniques. When placing new items on the shelves, you should put them behind the older products so that older products are used first. Reading labels to find storage information (choice 1), checking and marking inventory sheets (choice 2), and making notes about supplies that are running low (choice 3) are all examples of proper inventory-control techniques. Therefore, choices 1, 2, and 3 are incorrect.

200. **The correct answer is 2.** When an animal has been penetrated by a foreign body and the object is protruding from the animal, the object should be cut close to the wound. It shouldn't be removed before transporting the patient, however, so choice 4 is not correct. Choice 1 is incorrect because wounds should never be dressed using cotton or wool gauze, as the fabric may stick to the open wound. Choice 3 is incorrect because wounds should only be cleaned with antiseptic ointments that are soluble in water.

ANSWER SHEET PRACTICE TEST 3

1. ① ② ③ ④	41. ① ② ③ ④	81. ① ② ③ ④	121. ① ② ③ ④	161. ① ② ③ ④
2. ① ② ③ ④	42. ① ② ③ ④	82. ① ② ③ ④	122. ① ② ③ ④	162. ① ② ③ ④
3. ① ② ③ ④	43. ① ② ③ ④	83. ① ② ③ ④	123. ① ② ③ ④	163. ① ② ③ ④
4. ① ② ③ ④	44. ① ② ③ ④	84. ① ② ③ ④	124. ① ② ③ ④	164. ① ② ③ ④
5. ① ② ③ ④	45. ① ② ③ ④	85. ① ② ③ ④	125. ① ② ③ ④	165. ① ② ③ ④
6. ① ② ③ ④	46. ① ② ③ ④	86. ① ② ③ ④	126. ① ② ③ ④	166. ① ② ③ ④
7. ① ② ③ ④	47. ① ② ③ ④	87. ① ② ③ ④	127. ① ② ③ ④	167. ① ② ③ ④
8. ① ② ③ ④	48. ① ② ③ ④	88. ① ② ③ ④	128. ① ② ③ ④	168. ① ② ③ ④
9. ① ② ③ ④	49. ① ② ③ ④	89. ① ② ③ ④	129. ① ② ③ ④	169. ① ② ③ ④
10. ① ② ③ ④	50. ① ② ③ ④	90. ① ② ③ ④	130. ① ② ③ ④	170. ① ② ③ ④
11. ① ② ③ ④	51. ① ② ③ ④	91. ① ② ③ ④	131. ① ② ③ ④	171. ① ② ③ ④
12. ① ② ③ ④	52. ① ② ③ ④	92. ① ② ③ ④	132. ① ② ③ ④	172. ① ② ③ ④
13. ① ② ③ ④	53. ① ② ③ ④	93. ① ② ③ ④	133. ① ② ③ ④	173. ① ② ③ ④
14. ① ② ③ ④	54. ① ② ③ ④	94. ① ② ③ ④	134. ① ② ③ ④	174. ① ② ③ ④
15. ① ② ③ ④	55. ① ② ③ ④	95. ① ② ③ ④	135. ① ② ③ ④	175. ① ② ③ ④
16. ① ② ③ ④	56. ① ② ③ ④	96. ① ② ③ ④	136. ① ② ③ ④	176. ① ② ③ ④
17. ① ② ③ ④	57. ① ② ③ ④	97. ① ② ③ ④	137. ① ② ③ ④	177. ① ② ③ ④
18. ① ② ③ ④	58. ① ② ③ ④	98. ① ② ③ ④	138. ① ② ③ ④	178. ① ② ③ ④
19. ① ② ③ ④	59. ① ② ③ ④	99. ① ② ③ ④	139. ① ② ③ ④	179. ① ② ③ ④
20. ① ② ③ ④	60. ① ② ③ ④	100. ① ② ③ ④	140. ① ② ③ ④	180. ① ② ③ ④
21. ① ② ③ ④	61. ① ② ③ ④	101. ① ② ③ ④	141. ① ② ③ ④	181. ① ② ③ ④
22. ① ② ③ ④	62. ① ② ③ ④	102. ① ② ③ ④	142. ① ② ③ ④	182. ① ② ③ ④
23. ① ② ③ ④	63. ① ② ③ ④	103. ① ② ③ ④	143. ① ② ③ ④	183. ① ② ③ ④
24. ① ② ③ ④	64. ① ② ③ ④	104. ① ② ③ ④	144. ① ② ③ ④	184. ① ② ③ ④
25. ① ② ③ ④	65. ① ② ③ ④	105. ① ② ③ ④	145. ① ② ③ ④	185. ① ② ③ ④
26. ① ② ③ ④	66. ① ② ③ ④	106. ① ② ③ ④	146. ① ② ③ ④	186. ① ② ③ ④
27. ① ② ③ ④	67. ① ② ③ ④	107. ① ② ③ ④	147. ① ② ③ ④	187. ① ② ③ ④
28. ① ② ③ ④	68. ① ② ③ ④	108. ① ② ③ ④	148. ① ② ③ ④	188. ① ② ③ ④
29. ① ② ③ ④	69. ① ② ③ ④	109. ① ② ③ ④	149. ① ② ③ ④	189. ① ② ③ ④
30. ① ② ③ ④	70. ① ② ③ ④	110. ① ② ③ ④	150. ① ② ③ ④	190. ① ② ③ ④
31. ① ② ③ ④	71. ① ② ③ ④	111. ① ② ③ ④	151. ① ② ③ ④	191. ① ② ③ ④
32. ① ② ③ ④	72. ① ② ③ ④	112. ① ② ③ ④	152. ① ② ③ ④	192. ① ② ③ ④
33. ① ② ③ ④	73. ① ② ③ ④	113. ① ② ③ ④	153. ① ② ③ ④	193. ① ② ③ ④
34. ① ② ③ ④	74. ① ② ③ ④	114. ① ② ③ ④	154. ① ② ③ ④	194. ① ② ③ ④
35. ① ② ③ ④	75. ① ② ③ ④	115. ① ② ③ ④	155. ① ② ③ ④	195. ① ② ③ ④
36. ① ② ③ ④	76. ① ② ③ ④	116. ① ② ③ ④	156. ① ② ③ ④	196. ① ② ③ ④
37. ① ② ③ ④	77. ① ② ③ ④	117. ① ② ③ ④	157. ① ② ③ ④	197. ① ② ③ ④
38. ① ② ③ ④	78. ① ② ③ ④	118. ① ② ③ ④	158. ① ② ③ ④	198. ① ② ③ ④
39. ① ② ③ ④	79. ① ② ③ ④	119. ① ② ③ ④	159. ① ② ③ ④	199. ① ② ③ ④
40. ① ② ③ ④	80. ① ② ③ ④	120. ① ② ③ ④	160. ① ② ③ ④	200. ① ② ③ ④

Practice Test 3

1. Which of the following devices on a rebreathing anesthesia machine converts the liquid anesthetic to a gas state?
   1. Pressure reducing valve
   2. Vaporizer
   3. Oxygen flush valve
   4. Flowmeter

2. Which of the following is a type of radiation therapy that is implanted directly in the area to be treated?
   1. Brachytherapy
   2. Thoracoscopy
   3. Laparoscopy
   4. Radiofrequency ablation

3. A patient has been brought into the lobby of the veterinary office. When the animal is triaged you should check its:
   1. red blood cell count.
   2. pulse rate.
   3. white blood cell count.
   4. length.

4. Morphine is an example of which of the following classifications of drugs?
   1. Schedule I
   2. Schedule II
   3. Schedule IV
   4. Schedule V

5. Which of the following bandages is *most likely* used when wrapping the tail of an animal?
   1. Crepe
   2. Cohesive
   3. Tubular
   4. Open weave

6. All the following belong to the "triad of anesthesia" *except*:
   1. analgesia.
   2. muscle relaxation.
   3. consciousness.
   4. narcosis.

7. Which of the following would be considered biomedical waste?
   1. Plastic that is covered with the blood of a healthy rabbit
   2. Feces from a cat that is infected with ear mites
   3. Sponges that are soaked in the salvia of a dog with rabies
   4. Tissue from a castration on a healthy bovine

8. Which of the following is a fat-soluble vitamin?
   1. Folic acid
   2. C
   3. Biotin
   4. E

9. Which of the following statements is true regarding anesthesia during the dental prophylaxis?
   1. Anesthesia is only used on large dog breeds during the dental prophylaxis.
   2. Anesthesia is avoided during the dental prophylaxis.
   3. Anesthesia is needed to perform a dental radiograph.
   4. Anesthesia is only used on small animals during the dental prophylaxis.

10. Myelography is the radiographic examination of the:
    1. nerves.
    2. heart.
    3. spinal cord.
    4. brain.

11. The anesthetist announces that the patient's leg has been blocked. This means that the patient's leg:
    1. is unable to receive anesthesia.
    2. is broken or injured.
    3. has been operated on.
    4. was given local anesthetic.

12. All the following animals develop deciduous teeth *except*:
    1. cats.
    2. dolphins.
    3. sharks.
    4. cattle.

13. Which of the following is an example of a non-elective surgery?
    1. Spaying a 4-year-old cat
    2. Removing cataracts from a 14-year-old dog
    3. Docking the tail of a 3-day-old puppy
    4. Removing a tumor from a 6-year-old dog

14. A periodontal probe is used to:
    1. extract a tooth.
    2. scrape calculus.
    3. test tooth mobility.
    4. check for cavities.

15. A puppy's weight is made up of what percentage of water?
    1. 15%
    2. 40%
    3. 75%
    4. 80%

16. A small hole is discovered in the sterile sheet during the draping process, you should:
    1. cover the hole with a piece of sterile gauze.
    2. discard the sheet.
    3. fold the sheet so the hole is not noticeable.
    4. continue draping.

17. Which of the following is the *most* common cause of tooth loss in cats?
    1. Resorptive lesions
    2. Gingivitis
    3. Periodontal disease
    4. Stomatitis

18. How long should ruminants fast prior to surgery?
    1. 2–4 hours
    2. 6–12 hours
    3. 12–24 hours
    4. 24–48 hours

19. Which of the following stain methods is used to examine bacteria?
    1. Gram's
    2. Leishman's
    3. Wright's
    4. Sudan III

20. You are monitoring a cat that has already completely come out of anesthesia after surgery. The best place to monitor the cat's pulse is at its:
    1. cephalic vein.
    2. femoral artery.
    3. saphenous vein.
    4. lingual artery.

21. An important task of the veterinary technician is to manage the inventory of the office. Which of the following statements does *not* describe managing inventory?
    1. The veterinary technician keeps a list of frequently used items.
    2. The veterinary technician maintains a log of all the office's supplies.
    3. The veterinary technician purchases items the office needs.
    4. The veterinary technician organizes all the patient's medical files.

22. During surgery you notice that a dog's gums have turned a bluish color. Which of the following conditions could this represent?
    1. Methemoglobinemia
    2. Anemia
    3. Shock
    4. Cyanosis

23. All the following statements about esophagography are correct *except*:
    1. they require previous radiographs of the cervical region and thorax.
    2. they allow for assessment of esophageal motility.
    3. they require injured or ill animals to be anesthetized.
    4. they allow for an animal to eat bits of food to complete the test.

24. A dog's tail should be docked at:
    1. 2–5 days old.
    2. 2–5 weeks old.
    3. 2–5 months old.
    4. 2–5 years old.

25. One of the side effects of oxytetracycline is:
    1. skin rash.
    2. hyperactivity.
    3. discoloration of teeth.
    4. temporary blindness.

26. An intravenous catheter is placed during which of the following stages of anesthesia?
    1. First stage
    2. Second stage
    3. Third stage, plane 1
    4. Third stage, plane 3

27. All the following are side effects of radiation *except*:
    1. odor.
    2. hair loss.
    3. itchiness.
    4. hyperactivity.

28. Which of the following anesthetic drugs is inhaled?
    1. Isoflurane
    2. Thiopental
    3. Lidocaine
    4. Pentobarbital

29. When a gastrointestinal drug is administered, the part of the body that absorbs *most* of the drug is the:
    1. tongue.
    2. stomach.
    3. small intestine.
    4. large intestine.

30. An animal is anesthetized during all the following procedures *except*:
    1. radiation therapy.
    2. MRI scans.
    3. CAT scans.
    4. ultrasound exam.

31. Physical examinations should be performed starting with the:
    1. tail and ending at the nose.
    2. stomach and ending with the spine.
    3. nose and ending at the tail.
    4. front paws and ending with the back paws.

32. After a cat undergoes a tooth extraction, it should be given which of the following types of medications?
    1. Meclizine
    2. Carprofen
    3. Amitriptyline
    4. Verapamil

33. Which of the following surgeries repairs bones, joints, and muscles?
    1. Angioplasty
    2. Tonsillectomy
    3. Biopsy
    4. Orthopedic

34. In dogs, *bordetella bronchiseptica* causes:
    1. kennel cough.
    2. reovirus.
    3. diabetes.
    4. distemper.

35. Which of the following medications should be used to treat separation anxiety?
    1. Etodolac
    2. Clomipramine
    3. Deracoxib
    4. Carprofen

36. Sarcoptic mange is caused by:
    1. mites.
    2. fleas.
    3. ticks.
    4. mosquitoes.

37. Which of the following should be used to remove hair prior to surgery?
    1. Razors
    2. Clippers
    3. Depilatories
    4. Wax

38. Vetsulin is used to treat which of the following conditions in cats and dogs?
    1. Conjunctivitis
    2. Inflammation
    3. Cancer
    4. Diabetes

39. Surgical wound infection rates increase as the time period between hair removal and:
    1. surgery increases.
    2. anesthesia administration increases.
    3. surgery decreases.
    4. anesthesia administration decreases.

40. A cat with type A blood can receive:
    1. neither AB nor B blood.
    2. only AB blood.
    3. only B blood.
    4. both AB and B blood.

41. Night blindness in cattle is a common symptom of a deficiency of vitamin:
1. A.
2. D.
3. E.
4. K.

42. Which of the following is an advantage to using a rebreathing anesthesia machine?
1. More oxygen and anesthetic gases are used.
2. Depth of anesthesia can be changed more rapidly.
3. Less waste gases are produced.
4. Resistance occurs less often during respirations.

43. Newcastle disease *most* commonly affects:
1. humans.
2. poultry.
3. cattle.
4. frogs.

44. Luxating patella is a condition that affects a small dog's:
1. joints.
2. hip.
3. kneecap.
4. muscles.

45. The gestation period for a hog is usually:
1. 35–38 days.
2. 75–78 days.
3. 112–115 days.
4. 126–129 days.

46. All the following are common systemic fungal diseases *except*:
1. blastomycosis.
2. histoplasmosis.
3. coccidioidomycosis.
4. halitosis.

47. A dog weighs 11 pounds (5 kg) and requires a drug dose rate at 1 mg/kg. The solution is 0.5%. How many ml does the dog need?
1. 0.2 ml
2. 0.5 ml
3. 1 ml
4. 1.5 ml

48. Within one year of being diagnosed with diabetes, 75% of all dogs will develop:
1. cataracts.
2. cancer.
3. kidney infections.
4. hip dysplasia.

49. An Amazon parrot is brought to the veterinary clinic. Its owner says the bird is making a wheezing noise and is having trouble breathing. No discharge is coming from the bird's beak or nasal passages. What could be causing the symptoms?
1. Aspergillosis
2. Bronchitis
3. Enteritis
4. Scabies

50. Which of the following medications is used to prevent heartworm?
1. Atenolol
2. Ivermectin
3. Imidacloprid
4. Midazolam

51. The *most* common surgery in cats and dogs is:
1. spaying/neutering.
2. dental prophylaxis.
3. joint replacement.
4. tooth extraction.

52. An 8-month-old Rottweiler is diagnosed with severe hip dysplasia on his left side, but the joints have no damage. Which of the following surgeries should be used to treat the condition?
1. Femoral head and neck excision
2. Total hip replacement
3. Juvenile pubic symphysiodesis
4. Triple pelvic osteotomy

53. All the following are reasons why veterinarians and technicians perform patient assessments *except*:
1. patient assessments establish a baseline of the animal's health.
2. patient assessments help owners decide if they wish to proceed with surgery.
3. patient assessments are general and can be performed on any type of animal.
4. patient assessments affect the surgical outcome and future health of the animal.

54. A 7-year-old male cat is brought into the veterinary office by his owner. The owner tells the vet that when his cat visits the litter box he meows but does not urinate. The cat has also stopped eating and is lethargic. After an examination, the veterinarian determines that the cat has a urinary blockage. Which of following should the veterinarian use to treat this condition?
    1. Exploratory surgery
    2. Perineal urethrostomy
    3. Cystocentesis
    4. Urohydropropulsion

55. Which of the following stances *most likely* indicates a dog is assertive and potentially aggressive?
    1. The dog has a relaxed face, and its ears move toward sound.
    2. The dog has its lips curled and teeth bared, and it maintains eye contact.
    3. The dog stays low to the ground, and its ears are flattened to the side.
    4. The dog avoids eye contact and has its ears back and down.

56. Which of the following conditions is *most likely* to be mistaken for normal aging?
    1. Ichthyosis
    2. Addison's disease
    3. Cushing's disease
    4. Gastritis

57. To prevent hypothermia in birds, small animals, and reptiles after surgery, they are:
    1. placed in an incubator.
    2. wrapped in wet towels.
    3. kept under anesthesia longer.
    4. woken up immediately after surgery.

58. An owner brings a 2-year-old mastiff to the veterinary office. The dog refuses to eat, but it is drinking and is active. The veterinary medical team examines the dog, runs blood tests, and performs an X-ray. All the results come back normal. The dog is put on an antidepressant and sent home with his owner. After two days, the dog is still not eating. The veterinary staff's next course of action should be:
    1. castration.
    2. exploratory surgery.
    3. perineal urethrostomy.
    4. juvenile pubic symphysiodesis.

59. Which of the following are used to treat ectoparasites on animals?
    1. Fipronil
    2. Sertraline
    3. Chlorambucil
    4. Meloxicam

60. Before the surgical procedure begins, the patient and surrounding areas are surrounded with a barrier to:
    1. maintain a sterile area during surgery.
    2. reduce the amount of cleaning after surgery.
    3. prevent hypothermia of the patient.
    4. protect the surgical team from infection.

61. All the following animals could undergo a cholecystectomy *except* a:
    1. horse.
    2. snake.
    3. dog.
    4. lizard.

62. *Dirofilaria immitis* is transmitted from host to host by:
    1. mosquitoes.
    2. fleas.
    3. ticks.
    4. humans.

63. When setting up the surgical station, you should use grasping forceps such as a hemostat to:
    1. open packs of surgical instruments.
    2. trim pieces of gauze.
    3. pick up surgical instruments.
    4. connect tubing to machines.

64. An owner brings her 4-month-old male ferret to the veterinary office because of a rancid smell coming from the animal. She has bathed him and the animal still smells. The veterinarian examines the ferret and does not find anything wrong with it. What should the veterinarian do to rectify this problem?
    1. Neuter the ferret.
    2. Descent the ferret.
    3. Bathe the ferret.
    4. Euthanatize the ferret.

65. A veterinarian has scheduled an operation in which he will make an incision in a cat's intestine. This procedure is called:
 1. laparotomy.
 2. enterotomy.
 3. colotomy.
 4. osteotomy.

66. All the following pieces of information should be recorded in the accident book following any type of accident *except* the:
 1. occupation of person who had the accident.
 2. name of person who had the accident.
 3. home address of person who had the accident.
 4. social security number of person who had the accident.

67. Why are cats difficult to intubate?
 1. Their larynx is prone to spasms.
 2. Their epiglottis is very small.
 3. Their epiglottis is prone to spasms.
 4. Their larynx is very large.

68. An autoclave sterilizes instruments with:
 1. soap and water.
 2. disinfectants.
 3. steam.
 4. heat.

69. A cat is diagnosed with kidney disease and must undergo surgery to remove one of its kidneys. Which of the following procedures will be performed on the cat?
 1. Lumpectomy
 2. Appendectomy
 3. Hysterectomy
 4. Nephrectomy

70. An adrenergic drug's pharmacologic effects imitate:
 1. sympathetic nervous system activity.
 2. cardiovascular system activity.
 3. skeletal system activity.
 4. lymphatic system activity.

71. Analgesics are used prior to surgery for:
 1. pain relief.
 2. sedation.
 3. muscle relaxation.
 4. anxiety.

72. All the following are used to close incisions after surgery *except*:
 1. absorbable sutures.
 2. tissue glue.
 3. staples.
 4. scalpel.

73. Which of the following conditions requires emergency surgery?
 1. Gastric dilation-volvulus
 2. Luxating patella
 3. Hip dysplasia
 4. Ovariohysterectomy

74. All the following animals need to fast prior to surgery *except*:
 1. birds.
 2. rats.
 3. cattle.
 4. dogs.

75. The procedure of covering a patient and surrounding areas with a sterile cotton, paper, or plastic sheet prior to a surgical procedure is called:
 1. toweling.
 2. draping.
 3. disinfecting.
 4. sterilization.

76. Which of the following instruments is used to initially remove thick calculus from an animal's teeth during the dental prophylaxis?
 1. Forceps
 2. Scaler
 3. Irrigation needle
 4. Periodontal probe

77. Sutures over joints should be removed in:
 1. 7 days.
 2. 10 days.
 3. 14 days.
 4. 21 days.

78. A veterinarian has scheduled an operation in which an incision will be made in a dog's bladder. This procedure is called:
 1. cystocentesis.
 2. pyometra.
 3. cystotomy.
 4. ovariohysterectomy.

79. Surgery is the best course of treatment for which of the following conditions?
    1. Aspergillosis
    2. Enteritis
    3. Newcastle disease
    4. Hepatic lipidosis

80. During the dental prophylaxis, it is important to apply the 10-second rule when using the scaler and polisher because these instruments can:
    1. scratch the tooth enamel.
    2. harm the gums.
    3. damage the root of the tooth.
    4. harm the tooth pulp with heat.

81. Which of the following is a symptom of onchocerciasis in horses?
    1. Lameness
    2. Wheezing
    3. Open sores
    4. Discolored feces

82. Which of the following instruments is used to help examine a guinea pig's teeth?
    1. Hobbles
    2. Buccal pad separators
    3. Hemostat
    4. Ophthalmoscope

83. After giving an injection to an 8-month-old cat, what should you do with the used needle?
    1. Flush it down the toilet.
    2. Dispose of it in a trash receptacle.
    3. Place it in a designated container.
    4. Sterilize it for reuse.

84. All the following are common dental procedures for animals except:
    1. root canal.
    2. dental prophylaxis.
    3. extraction.
    4. periapical.

85. Laboratory equipment should be sterilized by:
    1. using an autoclave.
    2. washing it in hot water.
    3. submerging it in alcohol.
    4. scrubbing it with antibacterial soap.

86. A rabbit is most likely to develop:
    1. pulpitis.
    2. malocclusion.
    3. gingivitis.
    4. plaque.

87. The condition in which a dog or cat is born with more teeth than normal is called:
    1. supernumerary.
    2. oligodontia.
    3. anodontia.
    4. deciduous.

88. Which of the following medications should be given to animals prior to anesthesia before the dental prophylaxis to prevent vomiting?
    1. Methocarbamol
    2. Amoxicillin
    3. Trifluridine
    4. Acepromazine

89. How many deciduous teeth does a horse have?
    1. 12
    2. 16
    3. 24
    4. 36

90. What is a Pasteur pipette used for in laboratories?
    1. To disinfect instruments
    2. To transfer liquids
    3. To clean wounds
    4. To pick up other instruments

91. All lab equipment and work surfaces should be cleaned:
    1. daily.
    2. weekly.
    3. biweekly.
    4. monthly.

92. All the following statements about fecal samples are true except:
    1. samples can be contaminated by grass.
    2. samples should be stored in an airtight container.
    3. samples can be contaminated by soil.
    4. samples should be stored at room temperature.

93. Smears should be dried by:
    1. a fan.
    2. a heater.
    3. the air.
    4. your breath.

94. Intravenous anesthesia should be administered to a pig in veins located in its:
    1. hoof.
    2. neck.
    3. snout.
    4. ear.

95. You open a cabinet containing chemicals, acids, and reagents. Which of the following do you see?
    1. Short clear and amber bottles
    2. Tall, thin bottles
    3. Dark green bottles
    4. Plastic bottles with snap-off caps

96. Which of the following animals are *most* prone to platelet clumping?
    1. Horses
    2. Birds
    3. Cats
    4. Lizards

97. After staining, basophilic cells will turn:
    1. red.
    2. orange.
    3. green.
    4. blue.

98. Which of the following medications is used as an anticoagulant?
    1. Idoxuridine
    2. Heparin
    3. Enalapril
    4. Praziquantel

99. You are cleaning up the laboratory for the evening. Which of the following should be used to clean the lenses of a microscope?
    1. Disinfectant solutions
    2. Lens paper
    3. Soap and water
    4. Autoclave

100. Blood samples are usually taken from a rabbit's:
    1. ears.
    2. tail.
    3. feet.
    4. neck.

101. When injecting a dog in the external jugular vein, it is important to avoid hitting the:
    1. carotid artery.
    2. cephalic vein.
    3. femoral artery.
    4. saphenous vein.

102. Which of the following describes why a fecal specimen bottle should be labeled on its side and *not* on its lid?
    1. Labels on lids can be more easily removed than labels on containers.
    2. If you remove the labeled lid, the specimen is no longer labeled.
    3. Specimen containers look more professional with labels on the side.
    4. Fecal specimens don't need lids, so it's pointless to label a lid.

103. Crenation causes red blood cells to:
    1. divide.
    2. mutate.
    3. expand.
    4. shrink.

104. The veterinary medical team suspects a dog has been poisoned by carbon monoxide. To perform a toxicology screening, which of the following samples should you collect?
    1. Whole blood
    2. Urine
    3. Serum
    4. Stomach contents

105. The inability to pass urine is called:
    1. pyometra.
    2. anuria.
    3. hematuria.
    4. polydipsia.

106. Which of the following is *most likely* to damage a whole blood sample?
    1. Storing the sample in a cold area
    2. Inverting or rolling the sample tube
    3. Using a wide-gauge needle for collection
    4. Exposing the sample to full sunlight

107. The average weight of a female adult golden retriever is:
    1. 5–10 pounds.
    2. 30–40 pounds.
    3. 60–70 pounds.
    4. 90–100 pounds.

108. Which of the following would make the best urine collection container?
    1. A clear plastic container with a snap-on lid
    2. An opaque plastic container with a screw-on lid
    3. A clear plastic container with a screw-on lid
    4. An opaque plastic container with a snap-on lid

109. The average life expectancy for a ferret is:
    1. 1–2 years.
    2. 3–4 years.
    3. 5–7 years
    4. 12–15 years

110. Rabies is spread through:
    1. saliva.
    2. blood.
    3. urine.
    4. feces.

111. When is the best time to collect a voided urine sample?
    1. Right after the patient wakes up
    2. Just after the patient eats
    3. Right before the patient eats
    4. Just before the patient goes to sleep

112. A common symptom of colitis is:
    1. inability to produce urine.
    2. diarrhea.
    3. constipation.
    4. inability to regurgitate.

113. If you are collecting multiple blood specimens from the same patient, the first samples you should collect are:
    1. blood culture tubes.
    2. heparin tubes.
    3. EDTA tubes.
    4. anticoagulation-free tubes.

114. Coprophagia is the practice of eating:
    1. rocks.
    2. feces.
    3. grass.
    4. trash.

115. A Yorkshire terrier is attacked by a German shepherd while out on a walk with its owner. The dog is unconscious and hemorrhaging from his left paw and left ear. This is an example of which type of emergency?
    1. Life-threatening
    2. Serious
    3. Minor
    4. Nonemergency

116. Which of the following types of wounds has jagged, uneven edges?
    1. Abrasion
    2. Laceration
    3. Puncture
    4. Contusion

117. During which of the following planes of the third stage of anesthesia is the animal still able to blink and swallow?
    1. Plane 1
    2. Plane 2
    3. Plane 3
    4. Plane 4

118. When packing blood samples to go to a laboratory, you should make sure that whole blood samples are:
    1. not directly touching ice packs.
    2. placed directly beside an ice pack.
    3. not refrigerated or put in a cooler.
    4. put between two pieces of dry ice.

119. Forceps are used for all the following functions *except* to:
    1. grasp and hold tissue.
    2. pick up surgical instruments.
    3. remove calculus from teeth.
    4. cut through sutures.

120. All the following are able to mail pathological specimens *except*:
    1. universities.
    2. dental practices.
    3. veterinary practices.
    4. laboratories.

121. A patient needs a blood sample taken through venipuncture. Before you take the sample, you should occlude the proximal part of the vein so that the:
    1. vein is easier to see and identify.
    2. area around the vein becomes numb.
    3. patient becomes more relaxed.
    4. injection site does not bleed excessively.

122. Which of the following catheters is used only for cats?
    1. Tieman's
    2. Jackson
    3. Foley
    4. Robinson

123. All the following have urinary bladders *except*:
    1. cats.
    2. snakes.
    3. ferrets.
    4. cattle.

124. Which of the following is an example of a topical medication?
    1. Lincomycin
    2. Imidacloprid
    3. Xylazine
    4. Nitroprusside

125. A patient needs cells taken from the ear canal. The best instruments to collect such samples are:
    1. low-gauge needles.
    2. scalpels.
    3. cotton swabs.
    4. forceps.

126. Which of these is nontoxic to dogs?
    1. antifreeze.
    2. cocoa mulch.
    3. azaleas.
    4. chestnuts.

127. Which of the following is a symptom of dehydration?
    1. Dry eyes
    2. Dry gums
    3. Dry hair
    4. Dry skin

128. An example of an animal with brachydont teeth is a:
    1. rabbit.
    2. horse.
    3. deer.
    4. cat.

129. How many different canine blood groups exist?
    1. 3
    2. 5
    3. 8
    4. 10

130. Which of the following is a common cause of pyrexia (or high body temperature)?
    1. General anesthesia
    2. Shock
    3. Circulatory collapse
    4. Infection

131. A dog has ingested a toxic plant and is now unconscious. Why should you avoid treating the dog with emetics?
    1. Dogs should never be treated with emetics.
    2. Emetics should only be given if the patient is having seizures.
    3. Unconscious animals shouldn't be treated with emetics.
    4. Patients shouldn't be given emetics if they eat toxic plants.

132. The veterinarian decides to close a patient's wound four days after a patient arrives at the clinic with injuries from a car accident. The veterinarian decides to wait this long so contaminants come out of the wound before it's sutured. Which type of wound closure did the veterinarian use?
    1. Primary closure
    2. Delayed primary closure
    3. Tertiary closure
    4. Secondary closure

133. A patient has been admitted to your clinic with an infectious disease and is put in isolation to keep other patients safe. Which of the following actions should you *avoid* when dealing with the infected patient?
    1. Placing the patient's chart outside its room
    2. Wearing disposable gloves when handling the patient
    3. Tending to the infected patient before other patients
    4. Disposing of the patient's needles in the biomedical waste

134. Which of the following is a common reason for non-healing wounds?
    1. The sutures are placed too close to the edge of the wound.
    2. Circulation at the site of the wound has increased.
    3. Absorbable sutures are left on the wound for an extended period.
    4. Too little moisture accumulates at the wound after closure.

135. The veterinarian has a note on a patient's chart that says the patient should be administered a drug "PO t.i.d." What does the veterinarian's note mean?
    1. The patient should get the drug by mouth three times per day.
    2. The patient should get the drug by mouth four times per day.
    3. The patient should get the drug intravenously three times per day.
    4. The patient should get the drug intravenously four times per day.

136. A dog comes to your clinic with a puncture wound. Which of the following incidents would *most likely* cause a puncture wound?
    1. Excessive head shaking
    2. Exposure to broken glass
    3. A road or traffic accident
    4. Contact with a fish hook

137. All the following are stages of mitosis *except*:
    1. prophase.
    2. metaphase.
    3. interphase.
    4. anaphase.

138. The study of the tissues of the body is called:
    1. anatomy.
    2. histology.
    3. physiology
    4. pathology.

139. An 8-week-old puppy is brought to the veterinary's office after being hit by a car. The puppy is not responding to the veterinarian, and the veterinarian orders a scan of the brain. Which of the following tests is used to examine the brain?
    1. CAT scan
    2. Endoscopy
    3. Ultrasound
    4. Rhinoscopy

140. A scalpel is used to:
    1. cut through sutures.
    2. close up wounds.
    3. make cuts in the skin.
    4. grasp and hold tissues.

141. What color are *most* oxygen tanks?
    1. Blue
    2. Green
    3. Red
    4. Orange

142. An ophthalmoscope is an instrument used to examine the:
    1. ears.
    2. mouth.
    3. heart.
    4. eyes.

143. While placing the instruments on the tray prior to surgery, you accidentally drop one on the floor. Which of the following steps should you do next?
    1. Replace it with a sterile instrument.
    2. Place it back on the tray.
    3. Wash it in the sink.
    4. Soak it in alcohol.

144. Which of the following is the best course of treatment for cataracts in animals?
    1. Scraping the conjunctiva
    2. Surgical removal of the lens of the affected eye or eyes
    3. Medicated eye drops
    4. Surgical removal of the affected eye or eyes

145. The veterinarian left a note about a patient that gives the orders "NPO." What do the veterinarian's orders mean?
   1. Give the animal nothing to eat or drink.
   2. Allow the animal to drink water but not to eat.
   3. Feed the animal as frequently as possible.
   4. Give the animal a limited amount of food and water.

146. Which part of the skeletal system is most visible on radiographs?
   1. Mineralized components
   2. Articular cartilage
   3. Osteoid matrix
   4. Lesions

147. All the following injuries typically require bandaging *except*:
   1. contusions.
   2. abrasions.
   3. lacerations.
   4. punctures.

148. When cleaning a patient's kennel, you should:
   1. move the patient to another animal's kennel.
   2. remove bedding but keep food bowls in place.
   3. rinse detergent and disinfectant thoroughly.
   4. allow the kennel to air dry after it is clean.

149. Nuclear tests are usually accompanied by a radioactive dye that is administered intravenously. This radioactive dye is administered intravenously, which means it is injected into the bloodstream through the:
   1. arteries.
   2. veins.
   3. capillaries.
   4. arterioles.

150. Which of the following disinfectants would *most likely* be used on skin?
   1. Bleach
   2. Triclosan
   3. Formaldehyde
   4. Ammonia

151. The surgical scrub you perform before surgeries should:
   1. be done with scalding hot water.
   2. last between 30 and 60 seconds.
   3. be completed with jewelry on.
   4. include your hands and forearms.

152. Which of the following is an example of an unethical act?
   1. Disposing of used needles in properly marked containers.
   2. Explaining medication doses to the animal's owner.
   3. Not documenting a minor chemical spill in the accident book.
   4. Forgetting to place a heating pad under an animal prior to surgery.

153. You are helping to administer a catheter into the vein of a dehydrated patient. Which of these steps should occur first?
   1. Clip the patient's fur.
   2. Tape the catheter to the patient's body.
   3. Disinfect the patient's skin.
   4. Occlude the vein to make it bulge.

154. Nuclear scintigraphy is *most* commonly used on horses to examine the function of:
   1. muscles.
   2. bones.
   3. ears.
   4. eyes.

155. Radiation is used to treat:
   1. tumors.
   2. bronchitis.
   3. osteoarthritis.
   4. urinary tract infections.

156. The purpose of the endotracheal tube on both the non-rebreathing anesthesia machine and rebreathing anesthesia machine is to carry gases:
   1. to the animal.
   2. to the lungs.
   3. from the animal.
   4. from the anesthetic machine.

157. A 4-year-old cat has had repeated urinary tract infections. The veterinarian orders a nuclear scan of the kidneys. Which of the following is the name for this type of test?
   1. Renal scintigraphy
   2. Ultrasound
   3. Cystocentesis
   4. Urine analysis

158. A noninvasive technique for diagnosing portosystemic shunts in dogs and cats is called:
1. renal scintigraphy.
2. thyroid scintigraphy.
3. portal scintigraphy.
4. brain scintigraphy.

159. Which of the following tests should be performed prior to a bone scintigraphy?
1. PET scan
2. X-ray
3. CAT scan
4. MRI

160. Local anesthetics help diagnose lameness in:
1. pigs.
2. cattle.
3. horses.
4. sheep.

161. Which of the following animals is a good candidate for an MRI?
1. 11-year-old golden retriever with a pacemaker
2. 3-month-old puppy with a microchip
3. 9-month-old pregnant ferret with a cloth bandage
4. 4-year-old rabbit with a BB pellet in its stomach

162. All the following statements about rebreathing anesthesia machines are true *except*:
1. they allow recirculation of exhaled gases to the animal.
2. they use a flowmeter to adjust the flow of oxygen to the animal.
3. they are used on animals weighing less than 10 pounds.
4. they include a reservoir bag that collects fresh and expired gas.

163. An ultrasound is used to help diagnose which of the following conditions?
1. Pregnancy
2. Luxating patella
3. Bone fracture
4. Hip dysplasia

164. During the second stage of anesthesia:
1. the animal is placed in an unconscious state.
2. surgery is performed on the animal.

3. the animal is monitored until it wakes.
4. medications are given to relax the animal.

165. Which of the following plants is nontoxic to cats?
1. Alfalfa
2. Baby's breath
3. Bamboo
4. Juniper

166. All the following are normal reactions from anesthesia *except*:
1. shivering.
2. vomiting.
3. urination.
4. dehydration.

167. Assisted ventilation must be used during which of the following planes of the third stage of anesthesia?
1. Planes 1 and 2
2. Planes 2 and 3
3. Planes 3 and 4
4. Planes 1 and 3

168. Which of the following patients should be moved only with the use of a stretcher?
1. A dog is collapsed with abdominal injuries
2. A cat is vomiting after ingesting a toxic plant
3. A dog is limping from a broken leg
4. A cat is bleeding after a fight with another animal

169. One way to test capillary refill time is to:
1. monitor the patient's pulse rate.
2. take the patient's blood pressure.
3. check the patient's temperature.
4. press on the patient's limb.

170. Which of the following is done as part of the preanesthetic screening process?
1. The animal is given blood tests.
2. The animal fasts for 12 hours.
3. The animal is given antibiotics.
4. The animal is given antianxiety medication.

171. Which of the following is part of a compound microscope's nosepiece?
1. Stage
2. Rheostat
3. Rotating turret
4. Optical tube

172. All the following are used to monitor the patient's heart rate and rhythm during anesthesia *except* a/ an:
1. stethoscope.
2. hand.
3. electrocardiogram.
4. ventilator

173. It is most difficult to place an endotracheal tube on which of the following animals?
1. Siamese cat
2. Akita dog
3. Persian cat
4. German shepherd dog

174. The abbreviation ADME stands for:
1. atrophy, distribution, metabolism, and elimination.
2. absorption, diet, metabolism, and excretion.
3. atrophy, distribution, medicine, and excretion.
4. absorption, distribution, metabolism, and elimination.

175. Anesthesia can cause all the following in an overweight dog *except*:
1. cardiac arrest.
2. prolonged time under anesthesia.
3. bladder problems.
4. liver problems.

176. Which of the following laryngoscope blades are curved?
1. Miller
2. Wisconsin
3. Phillips
4. Macintosh

177. When performing an endotracheal intubation on a dog, which of the following steps should you do first?
1. Check for air leakage.
2. Insert the tube.
3. Pull out the tongue.
4. Tape the tube in place.

178. Which of the following is true about patients' bandages?
1. Bandages on limbs should cover only the affected part of the limbs.
2. Wet or soiled bandages should be removed and replaced with dry bandages.
3. Bandages are loose if you can fit your finger between the bandage and the skin.
4. Pressure bandages should be removed 24 hours after you apply them.

179. After the endotracheal tube is placed in an animal, which of the following should be done next?
1. The cuff should be deflated.
2. The patient should be moved into position.
3. The cuff should be inflated.
4. The patient should be anesthetized.

180. Which of the following types of tablets can be divided?
1. Scored
2. Soft gelatin
3. Layered
4. Hard gelatin

181. Which of the following is *not* a part of a non-rebreathing anesthesia machine?
1. Endotracheal tube
2. Oxygen flush valve
3. Pressure reducing valve
4. Flowmeter

182. An animal that develops only one set of teeth is known as a:
1. monophyodont.
2. hypsodont.
3. diphyodont.
4. brachydont.

183. Special consideration should be paid when choosing how to anesthetize bovines, pigs, and goats because:
1. they need much higher doses than animals such as horses and dogs.
2. their owners generally do not want these animals to undergo surgery.
3. they are much more sensitive to anesthesia than other animals.
4. their meat and milk could be contaminated by the drugs.

184. Aminoglycosides are derived from bacteria of which genus?
    1. *Borrelia*
    2. *Streptomyces*
    3. *Thermotoga*
    4. *Leptospira*

185. All the following prevent periodontal disease in dogs *except*:
    1. daily tooth brushing.
    2. diet.
    3. chewing on bones.
    4. exercise.

186. Which of the following medications is given prior to anesthesia to help control the nervous system?
    1. Griseofulvin
    2. Diazepam
    3. Atropine
    4. Erythromycin

187. To test the pupillary reflex during anesthesia, you should:
    1. shine a light into the patient's eye.
    2. touch the corner of the patient's eye.
    3. pull gently on one of the patient's limbs.
    4. stimulate the patient's larynx.

188. While you're cutting a macaw's nails, you accidentally clip too close to the nail bed and the nail begins to bleed. Which of the following should you use to control the bleeding?
    1. Ketamine
    2. Meperidine
    3. St. John's Wort
    4. Styptic powder

189. Which of the following is the first step in preparing the surgery table for the surgeon?
    1. Adjust the table's height to the surgeon's preferences.
    2. Disinfect the table using a disinfectant spray.
    3. Place a heating blanket on the table.
    4. Perform the draping process.

190. Anesthesia has the fastest effect when it is administered:
    1. subcutaneously.
    2. intramuscularly.
    3. transdermally.
    4. intravenously.

191. Horses use their lips to grasp food and pull it into their mouths to eat. Because of these abilities, the lips are categorized as:
    1. lingual surfaces.
    2. prehensile organs.
    3. upper arcades.
    4. longitudinal muscles.

192. All the following are treatments for closed wounds *except*:
    1. pain medication.
    2. bandaging the wound.
    3. applying a splint.
    4. cold compresses.

193. Which of the following is a nuclear test that traces the path of an intravenous injection to diagnose or treat disease, cancer, or any other abnormality?
    1. CAT scan
    2. PET scan
    3. MRI
    4. Myelography

194. Lidocaine is an example of a:
    1. local anesthetic.
    2. sedative.
    3. general anesthetic.
    4. fever reducer.

195. A dog can contract parvovirus by coming into contact with:
    1. infected fecal matter.
    2. contaminated water.
    3. sick humans.
    4. spoiled food.

196. A lavender Vacutainer with a pink collecting pot indicates a sample of whole blood and an anticoagulant of:
    1. EDTA.
    2. heparin.
    3. sodium citrate.
    4. oxalate fluoride.

197. What is the main purpose of the anesthesia machine?
    1. To keep the animal alive during surgery
    2. To deliver oxygen and anesthetic gas to the animal
    3. To monitor the effects of anesthesia on the animal
    4. To help the animal breathe while under anesthesia

198. Why should a heating pad be placed under the patient during surgery?
    1. To help keep the patient comfortable
    2. To maintain the patient's body temperature
    3. To regulate the patient's blood pressure
    4. To decrease the risk of infection

199. Which of the following medications is used to block pain sensation and prevent movement during surgery?
    1. Diazepam
    2. Bupivacaine
    3. Ketamine
    4. Midazolam

200. A dog weighing 30 pounds (13.6 kg) requires a drug dose rate at 10 mg/kg. It is available in a 2.0% solution. How many ml should you give the dog?
    1. 0.6 ml
    2. 6.8 ml
    3. 13.6 ml
    4. 136 ml

PRACTICE TEST 3: ANSWER KEY AND EXPLANATIONS

1. 2	41. 1	81. 3	121. 1	161. 3
2. 1	42. 3	82. 2	122. 2	162. 3
3. 2	43. 2	83. 3	123. 2	163. 1
4. 2	44. 3	84. 4	124. 2	164. 1
5. 3	45. 3	85. 1	125. 3	165. 3
6. 3	46. 4	86. 2	126. 4	166. 4
7. 3	47. 3	87. 1	127. 2	167. 3
8. 4	48. 1	88. 4	128. 4	168. 1
9. 3	49. 1	89. 3	129. 3	169. 4
10. 3	50. 2	90. 2	130. 4	170. 1
11. 4	51. 1	91. 1	131. 3	171. 3
12. 2	52. 4	92. 4	132. 2	172. 4
13. 4	53. 3	93. 3	133. 3	173. 3
14. 3	54. 2	94. 4	134. 1	174. 4
15. 4	55. 2	95. 1	135. 1	175. 3
16. 2	56. 3	96. 3	136. 4	176. 4
17. 1	57. 1	97. 4	137. 3	177. 3
18. 4	58. 2	98. 2	138. 2	178. 2
19. 1	59. 1	99. 2	139. 1	179. 3
20. 2	60. 1	100. 1	140. 3	180. 1
21. 4	61. 1	101. 1	141. 2	181. 2
22. 4	62. 1	102. 2	142. 4	182. 1
23. 3	63. 3	103. 4	143. 1	183. 4
24. 1	64. 2	104. 1	144. 2	184. 2
25. 3	65. 2	105. 2	145. 1	185. 4
26. 1	66. 4	106. 4	146. 1	186. 3
27. 4	67. 1	107. 4	147. 1	187. 1
28. 1	68. 3	108. 2	148. 3	188. 4
29. 3	69. 4	109. 3	149. 2	189. 2
30. 4	70. 1	110. 1	150. 2	190. 4
31. 3	71. 1	111. 1	151. 4	191. 2
32. 2	72. 4	112. 2	152. 3	192. 3
33. 4	73. 1	113. 1	153. 1	193. 2
34. 1	74. 2	114. 2	154. 2	194. 1
35. 2	75. 2	115. 1	155. 1	195. 1
36. 1	76. 1	116. 2	156. 2	196. 1
37. 2	77. 3	117. 1	157. 1	197. 2
38. 4	78. 3	118. 1	158. 3	198. 2
39. 1	79. 1	119. 4	159. 2	199. 3
40. 1	80. 4	120. 1	160. 3	200. 2

1. **The correct answer is 2.** The vaporizer converts the anesthetic liquid to a gas and adds this gas to the oxygen flowing through the rebreathing anesthesia machine. Choice 1 reduces the pressure in the oxygen tank. Choice 3 increases the amount of oxygen and decreases the amount of anesthesia flowing to the animal. Choice 4 adjusts the flow of oxygen to the animal.

2. **The correct answer is 1.** Brachytherapy is a type of radiation therapy that implants radioactive sources directly into the source of cancer. This is most commonly used to treat thyroid adenomas in cats and nasal tumors in dogs. Choice 2 is incorrect because thoracoscopy is an examination of the chest cavity. Laparoscopy is an exam of the abdominal cavity that is performed through a small incision in the wall of the abdomen or the navel, so choice 3 is incorrect. Choice 4 is incorrect because radiofrequency ablation is a medical procedure that uses imaging techniques to guide a needle electrode into an area to relieve pain or destroy a cancerous tumor.

3. **The correct answer is 2.** When triaging an animal, you should check its pulse rate and other vital signs. Choices 1 and 3 are incorrect because triaging an animal occurs on first inspection, and it does not include taking blood samples. Generally, the length or height of animal is not important during triage, so choice 4 is incorrect.

4. **The correct answer is 2.** Some narcotics, stimulants, and depressants are classified as Schedule II drugs because they have a high potential for abuse by the user. These drugs, such as morphine or oxycodone (Percodan), are safe when used medically. Schedule I drugs have no safe medical uses and a high potential for abuse by the user. Some examples of Schedule I drugs are heroin, LSD, and PCP. Schedule IV and V drugs have less risk than Schedule II drugs and are safe when used medically. Some examples of Schedule IV and V drugs are diazepam (Valium), hydrocodone with acetaminophen (Vicodin), and alprazolam (Xanax).

5. **The correct answer is 3.** Because tubular bandaging has elasticity, it's used to wrap an animal's tail or limbs. Crepe bandaging is a washable bandage used for wrapping the head or thorax, so choice 1 is incorrect. Choice 2 is not correct because cohesive bandaging is a self-adhesive bandage that doesn't stick to skin or hair. Open weave bandaging is strong, but doesn't conform to the patient's body well, so choice 4 is incorrect.

6. **The correct answer is 3.** The triad of anesthesia consists of analgesia, muscle relaxation, and narcosis, or unconsciousness. If the triad contains unconsciousness, then choice 3, consciousness, is not part of the triad. Choices 1, 2, and 4 are incorrect because they are required during anesthesia.

7. **The correct answer is 3.** Waste in a veterinary clinic is most often considered biomedical waste when it is sharp (a needle or a scalpel) or when it is contaminated with blood or other bodily fluids of an animal that has a disease that can be contracted by humans. Sponges that are soaked in the saliva of a dog with rabies are biomedical waste because rabies can be contracted by humans. Choice 1 is incorrect because the rabbit is healthy. Feces from a cat that is infected with ear mites is incorrect because the feces are not infected with a disease that humans can contract. Tissue from a castration on a healthy bovine is incorrect because tissue from healthy animals is considered regular waste.

8. **The correct answer is 4.** Folic acid, Vitamin C, and biotin (choices 1, 2, and 3) are water-soluble vitamins, so these choices are incorrect. Vitamin E is a fat-soluble vitamin.

9. **The correct answer is 3.** Because animals are easier to control under anesthesia, it is used for a variety of reasons during the dental prophylaxis, such as when performing examinations, dental radiographs (X-rays), extractions, and cleanings. Choices 1 and 4 are incorrect because anesthesia is used on animals of all sizes. Choice 2 is incorrect because anesthesia is used to help control the animal during the dental prophylaxis.

10. **The correct answer is 3.** Myelography is the radiographic examination of the spinal cord. During this procedure, a dye is injected into the patient's spinal canal, and then the patient is X-rayed to determine if the spinal cord is injured. Myelography is not used to examine the nerves, heart, or brain, so choices 1, 2, and 4 are incorrect.

11. **The correct answer is 4.** The term *blocked* means that local anesthesia was given to a particular part of the body. Therefore, the anesthetist's announcement means the patient's leg was given local anesthetic. Choices 1, 2, and 3 are incorrect because the term *blocked* does not mean a body part is unable to receive anesthesia, is broken or injured, or has been operated on.

12. **The correct answer is 2.** Dolphins are considered monophyodont and only develop one set of teeth in their lifetime. Choices 1 and 4 are incorrect because cats and cattle are considered diphyodont because they develop two sets of teeth (deciduous and permanent) in their lifetimes. Sharks are considered polyphyodont because they develop many sets of teeth during their life, so choice 3 is incorrect.

13. **The correct answer is 4.** Nonelective surgery is performed to maintain life and quality of life, so removing a tumor from a 6-year-old dog is an example of a nonelective surgery. Choices 1, 2, and 3 are incorrect because these are examples of elective procedures, which are not medically detrimental to the patient if they are not performed.

14. **The correct answer is 3.** A periodontal probe is used to test tooth mobility (choice 3), measure pocket depths around a tooth, evaluate furcation lesions, and determine degree of gingivitis. Forceps are used to extract a tooth or scrape calculus from a tooth, so choices 1 and 2 are incorrect. Choice 4 is incorrect because a dental radiograph is used to check for cavities.

15. **The correct answer is 4.** While an adult dog's weight is made up of 50–60% water, a puppy's weight is mostly 80% water. Choices 1, 2, and 3 are incorrect because these choices are too low.

16. **The correct answer is 2.** If a sterile sheet is damaged or has a hole in it, it could become contaminated and should be discarded. To prevent contaminating the sheet, you should never cover the hole with a piece of sterile gauze, fold the sheet so the hole is not noticeable, or continue draping, so choices 1, 3, and 4 are incorrect.

17. **The correct answer is 1.** Although cats are prone to many diseases of the mouth, the most common cause of tooth loss is resorptive lesions. Resorptive lesions lead to the loss of tooth structure and usually begin on the enamel of the tooth near the gum line and then spread to the entire tooth resulting in tooth loss. Choices 2, 3, and 4 are incorrect. Gingivitis is a condition that afflicts the gums. Stomatitis is the inflammation of the oral mucous membranes at the back of the mouth. These conditions can lead to periodontal disease, which causes the inflammation of a tooth's deep supporting structures.

18. **The correct answer is 4.** A ruminant such as a sheep or goat should fast for 24–48 hours prior to surgery. Choices 1, 2, and 3 are incorrect because these choices represent too little time that these types of animals should fast.

19. **The correct answer is 1.** Gram's stain is used to differentiate between different types of bacteria. Leishman's stain and Wright's stain are used to differentiate between different blood cell types, so choices 2 and 3 are incorrect. Sudan III stain is used to differentiate between lipids, so choice 4 is incorrect.

20. **The correct answer is 2.** The best places to monitor animals' pulse rates are arteries that run close to the skin. The femoral artery is a good place to monitor pulse rates on cats and dogs, so choice 2 is correct. Choices 1 and 3 are incorrect because arteries, not veins, are the best vessels for finding pulse rates. Choice 4, the lingual artery, is incorrect because this artery is located under the animal's tongue, and generally is used to determine pulse rates when animals are under general anesthesia.

21. **The correct answer is 4.** Choice 4 is correct because inventory does not include the patient's medical files. Choices 1, 2, and 3 describe inventory management, so those are incorrect.

22. **The correct answer is 4.** If the patient's gums turn bluish during surgery, this could be a sign of cyanosis. Cyanosis indicates a lack of oxygen in the blood, and a patient having blue gums is an indicator of low oxygen levels. Bluish gums are not an indication of methemoglobinemia, anemia, or shock, so choices 1, 2, and 3 are incorrect.

23. **The correct answer is 3.** Animals are generally conscious and alert during esophagographies. Esophagographies test esophagus function; unconsciousness alters the ways in which the

esophagus works and doesn't allow for technicians to observe the quality of function. Choices 1, 2, and 4 are incorrect because esophagographies do require previous radiographs of the cervical region and thorax. They also allow for assessment of esophageal motility and sometimes, depending on the injury, illness, or animal in question, technicians instruct the animal to eat bits of food so they can track the food's progress through the animal's systems.

24. **The correct answer is 1.** Dogs should have their tails docked when they are 2–5 days old. Choices 2, 3, and 4 are incorrect because these time periods are too long to wait to have a dog's tail docked.

25. **The correct answer is 3.** Because oxytetracycline and other tetracyclines can discolor the teeth in young animals, it should not be administered to animals whose adult teeth have not fully erupted. While skin rash (choice 1), hyperactivity (choice 2), and temporary blindness (choice 3), are common side effects of certain other medications, they are not side effects of oxytetracycline.

26. **The correct answer is 1.** An intravenous catheter is placed during the first stage of anesthesia because it needs to be in place to deliver anesthetics, fluids, and emergency medications (if needed) prior to the second and third stages of anesthesia. Choices 2, 3, and 4 are incorrect because the intravenous catheter should be placed before the second and third stages.

27. **The correct answer is 4.** Radiation does not cause hyperactivity. It can, however, cause odor from the treatment site due to dying cells, hair loss, and itchiness, so choices 1, 2, and 3 are incorrect.

28. **The correct answer is 1.** Isoflurane is administered as an inhalant, so choice 1 is correct. Choices 2 and 4 are incorrect because thiopental and pentobarbital are barbiturates that are generally injected. Choice 3, lidocaine, is incorrect because it is a local anesthetic that is generally injected.

29. **The correct answer is 3.** When a gastrointestinal drug is administered, the part of the body that absorbs most of the drug is the small intestine. The small intestine has a lot of open space that can absorb the drug. Choices 1 and 2 are incorrect because the gastrointestinal drugs are mostly

absorbed after passing over the tongue (choice 1) and through the stomach (choice 2). Choice 3 is incorrect because gastrointestinal drugs are mostly absorbed before they reach the large intestine.

30. **The correct answer is 4.** Animals may need to be restrained or sedated during an ultrasound, but they generally do not need to be anesthetized during this procedure. An animal is anesthetized during radiation, a MRI, and a CAT scan because these tests can cause pain or discomfort, and the patient needs to stay as still as possible during these tests; therefore, choices 1, 2, and 3 are incorrect.

31. **The correct answer is 3.** Physical examinations should start with assessment of the nostrils and end at the tail. The stomach, spine, and front and back paws should be checked between examination of the animal's face and rear. Choices 1, 2, and 4 are incorrect because they don't follow the nose-to-tail order.

32. **The correct answer is 2.** Carprofen, which is used to relieve pain, inflammation, and fever, should be given to a cat after a tooth extraction. Choice 1 is incorrect because meclizine is an antihistamine used to prevent motion sickness. Choice 3 is incorrect because amitriptyline is used to treat behavior problems. Choice 4 is incorrect because verapamil is used to treat cardiac and vascular conditions.

33. **The correct answer is 4.** Orthopedic surgery repairs bones, joints, and muscles. Angioplasty is a surgical procedure used to widen blood vessels in the heart, so choice 1 is incorrect. Choice 2 is incorrect because tonsillectomy is a surgical procedure to remove the tonsils. A biopsy is the removal of tissue, cells, fluids, or masses from the body, so choice 3 is incorrect.

34. **The correct answer is 1.** *Bordetella bronchiseptica* is a strain of bacteria that causes an upper-respiratory condition known as kennel cough in dogs. *Bordetella bronchiseptica* does not cause reovirus, diabetes, or distemper, so choices 2, 3, and 4 are incorrect. Reovirus is transmitted through contact with infected feces or airborne virus particles. Diabetes is caused by many factors including poor diet and health. Distemper is transmitted through airborne virus particles.

35. The correct answer is 2. Clomipramine is used to treat separation anxiety in animals. Etodolac, deracoxib, and carprofen are used to relieve pain, not treat separation anxiety, so choices 1, 3, and 4 are incorrect.

36. The correct answer is 1. Sarcoptic mange is a skin disease caused by a *Sarcoptes scabiei* mite, which lives and breeds in the host's skin. Choices 2, 3, and 4 are incorrect because none of these choices cause sarcoptic mange. Fleas can cause tapeworms and allergic reactions, ticks can cause Lyme disease, and mosquitoes can cause heartworm.

37. The correct answer is 2. Clippers should be used to remove hair prior to surgery. While razors, depilatories, and wax are effective at removing hair, they cause more skin trauma compared to clippers. Since skin trauma increases the chances of infection, choices 1, 3, and 4 are incorrect.

38. The correct answer is 4. Vetsulin (porcine insulin zinc suspension) is insulin specifically used to treat cats and dogs with diabetes. This drug is not effective in treating conjunctivitis, inflammation, or cancer, so choices 1, 2, and 3 are not correct.

39. The correct answer is 1. Surgical wound infection rates increase as the time period between hair removal and surgery increases. Hair removal causes trauma to the skin and increases the chances of a surgical wound infection. Choices 2 and 4 are incorrect because the time between anesthesia and hair removal does not affect infection rates. Choice 3 is incorrect because rate does not increase if the time period decreases.

40. The correct answer is 1. A cat with type A blood can receive neither AB nor B blood. Cats with this blood type can receive only type A blood. Choices 2, 3, and 4 are incorrect because cats with type A blood cannot receive AB or B blood types.

41. The correct answer is 1. Night blindness in cattle is caused by low levels of vitamin A. Choices 2, 3, and 4 are incorrect because deficiencies of vitamins D, E, and K are not related to night blindness in cattle.

42. The correct answer is 3. One of the advantages to using a rebreathing anesthesia machine is that less waste gases are produced. Choice 1 is incorrect because it uses less oxygen and anesthetic gases.

Choices 2 and 4 are incorrect because a non-rebreathing anesthesia machine allows for rapid control of the depth of anesthesia and less resistance during respirations.

43. The correct answer is 2. Newcastle disease is a highly contagious disease that affects the respiratory system of poultry kept in unsanitary conditions. This condition has no cure. Newcastle disease rarely affects humans, cattle, or frogs, so choices 1, 3, and 4 are incorrect.

44. The correct answer is 3. Luxating patella (patellar luxation) is a condition in which a dog's kneecap slips out of place causing pain. It mostly affects small dog breeds such as the toy fox terrier or Maltese. This condition does not affect a dog's joints, hip, or muscles, so choices 1, 2, and 4 are incorrect.

45. The correct answer is 3. The normal gestation period for a hog is 112–115 days. Choices 1 and 2 are incorrect because these time periods are too short. Choice 4 is incorrect because this time period is too long.

46. The correct answer is 4. Blastomycosis, histoplasmosis, and coccidioidomycosis are systemic fungal diseases, while halitosis is a condition that causes bad breath. Therefore, choices 1, 2, and 3 are incorrect.

47. The correct answer is 3. Use the formula Dose = body weight × dosage / concentration of drug. To get the percentage solution into mg/ml, multiply by 10. Dose = 5 kg × 1 mg/kg / 0.5% × 10 mg/ml = 5 kg × 1 mg/kg / 5 mg/ml, so choice 3, 1 ml is correct. Choices 1 and 2 are incorrect because those doses are too low. Choice 4 is incorrect because that dose is too high.

48. The correct answer is 1. One of the most common complications of diabetes in dogs is the rapid onset of cataracts. Cancer, kidney infections, and hip dysplasia are not generally caused by diabetes, so choices 2, 3, and 4 are incorrect.

49. The correct answer is 1. The Amazon is most likely suffering from aspergillosis, which is caused by a fungus that infects the bird's throat and lungs. It is usually caused by feeding a bird moldy bird seed. Bronchitis, which affects a bird's respiratory system, causes a nasal discharge and the bird to fluff its feathers more than usual, so choice 2 is incorrect. Choice 3 is incorrect because enteritis is an inflammation of the intestines caused by feeding a bird too much fruit or vegetables. Scabies is caused by a parasitic mite that usually gathers around the beak and legs, so choice 4 is incorrect.

50. **The correct answer is 2.** Ivermectin is used to prevent heartworm. Atenolol is a cardiac used to control heart rate and lower blood pressure, so choice 1 is incorrect. Choice 3 is incorrect because imidacloprid is a topical medication used to treat ectoparasites such as fleas or ticks. Midazolam is a sedative, so choice 4 is not correct.

51. **The correct answer is 1.** Spaying/neutering, which is the process of removing all or part of the animal's reproductive organs, is the most common surgery in cats and dogs. While dental prophylaxis, joint replacement, and tooth extraction are all common surgeries, these are not so common as spaying or neutering. Therefore, choices 2, 3, and 4 are incorrect.

52. **The correct answer is 4.** Triple pelvic osteotomy is the correct procedure to treat a dog that is 8 to 18 months old with hip dysplasia and no joint damage. Choice 1 is incorrect because femoral head and neck excision is performed on smaller breeds of dogs weighing less than 50 pounds. Choice 2 is incorrect because a total hip replacement is recommended for dogs with degenerative joint disease. Choice 3 is incorrect because juvenile pubic symphysiodesis is performed on puppies under the age of 5 months old.

53. **The correct answer is 3.** Veterinarians and technicians assess patients differently depending on the injury or disease, the patient's history, and the breed or species of the animal. Emergency conditions also affect the way veterinarians and technicians assess patients. Choices 1, 2, and 4 are reasons why veterinarians and technicians perform patient assessments.

54. **The correct answer is 2.** A perineal urethrostomy creates a new opening through which urine can pass and is performed on male cats with severe urinary blockages. Choice 1 is incorrect because the veterinarian does not need to perform exploratory surgery because he knows what is wrong with the cat. Choice 3 is incorrect because cystocentesis is a procedure in which a needle is inserted into the bladder to collect a urine sample. Choice 4 is incorrect because urohydropropulsion is a procedure used to help pass bladder stones through the urethra.

55. **The correct answer is 2.** If the dog has its lips curled and teeth bared, and it maintains eye contact, it is most likely assertive and potentially aggressive. Choice 1 is incorrect because a dog with a relaxed face and with ears that point toward sound is a relaxed dog. Choices 3 and 4 are incorrect because these dogs are most likely frightened, not assertive.

56. **The correct answer is 3.** Cushing's disease (hyperadrenocorticism) is a common condition in dogs that causes weight gain, hair loss, and diuresis—all of which could be mistaken for the normal aging process. It is caused by an increase in corticosteroid secretion from the adrenal gland. Choices 1, 2, and 4 are incorrect because they are not conditions that could be easily mistaken for normal aging. Ichthyosis is a hereditary condition that affects the eyes and skin. Addison's disease causes atrophy of the adrenal gland. Gastritis is caused by the inflammation of the lining of the stomach, usually caused by ingesting spoiled or contaminated foods, foreign objects, toxic plants, or chemicals.

57. **The correct answer is 1.** Birds, small animals, and reptiles should be placed in an incubator to prevent them from becoming hypothermic. Choice 2 is incorrect because a wet towel will not help to warm an animal. Choices 3 and 4 are incorrect because these changes in the amount of and timing of anesthesia will not make the animal warmer.

58. **The correct answer is 2.** Because the veterinarian is unsure of what is causing the dog to refuse food, the best course of action is exploratory surgery. Exploratory surgery is a diagnostic procedure to help determine what is wrong with an animal when all other avenues of treatment are exhausted. Castration, choice 1, the removal of a male dog's testicles, is incorrect because this procedure will do nothing to help find the source of dog's problem. Perineal urethrostomy is a procedure for male cats that creates a new opening through which urine can pass, so choice 3 is incorrect. Choice 4 is incorrect because juvenile pubic symphysiodesis

is a procedure performed on puppies less than 5 months old with hip dysplasia.

59. **The correct answer is 1.** Fipronil is a topical medication used to treat ectoparasites such as fleas and ticks. Sertraline is an antidepressant used to treat behavioral disorders, so choice 2 is not correct. Choice 3 is incorrect because chlorambucil is a medication used to treat blood cancer, lymphoma, and immune system conditions. Meloxicam is a nonsteroidal anti-inflammatory drug used to reduce pain, inflammation, and fever, so choice 4 is not correct.

60. **The correct answer is 1.** A barrier such as a cotton, paper, or plastic sheet is placed around the patient to maintain a sterile area during surgery. Choice 2 is not correct because barriers are not used to reduce the amount of the cleaning that needs to be done. Choice 3 is incorrect because it is not used to prevent hypothermia of the patient. Choice 4 is incorrect because the barrier is not used to prevent spreading infection to the surgical team.

61. **The correct answer is 1.** A cholecystectomy is the procedure in which the gallbladder is removed. It would not be performed on a horse because a horse does not have a gallbladder. A snake, dog, and lizard have gallbladders and, if needed, a cholecystectomy could be performed on any of these animals. Therefore, choices 2, 3, and 4 are incorrect.

62. **The correct answer is 1.** *Dirofilaria immitis*, or canine heartworm, is a parasite which infects a host by way of a mosquito bite. Heartworm is a serious condition that afflicts animals such as dogs, cats, wolves, coyotes, and foxes. *Dirofilaria immitis* is not transmitted by fleas, ticks, or humans, so choices 2, 3, and 4 are incorrect.

63. **The correct answer is 3.** Since the instruments are sterile, you should not use anything but grasping forceps to touch them or the instruments will be contaminated. Choices 1 and 2 are incorrect because grasping forceps should not be used to open packs of surgical instruments or trim pieces of gauze because this can contaminate these items. Choice 4 is incorrect because you shouldn't use forceps to connect tubing to machines.

64. **The correct answer is 2.** Ferrets have musk-producing glands on both sides of their anal opening that release an unpleasant odor when the animal feels threatened. Some ferrets secrete this odor all the time and a surgical procedure called descenting, which removes the ferret's anal sacs, is necessary to rid the animal of the odor. Choice 1 is incorrect because neutering the ferret will not affect the odor-producing anal sacs. Choice 3 is incorrect because bathing will not stop the ferret from producing the odor. Choice 4 is incorrect because the animal's condition does not warrant euthanasia.

65. **The correct answer is 2.** Enterotomy is a surgical procedure in which an incision is made in the intestine. Choice 1 is incorrect because a laparotomy is a procedure in which an incision is made in the abdomen. A colostomy is a procedure in which an incision is made in the colon, so choice 3 is incorrect. Choice 4 is incorrect because an osteotomy is a procedure in which the surgeon cuts into the bone.

66. **The correct answer is 4.** It's unnecessary to record the social security number of person who had the accident in the accident book. The occupation, name, and home address of the person who had the accident should be recorded in the accident book following the accident, so choices 1, 2, and 3 are incorrect.

67. **The correct answer is 1.** Because a cat's larynx is prone to spasms, veterinary technicians should use a small amount of a local anesthetic when placing the endotracheal tube. Choices 2, 3, and 4 are incorrect because these are not reasons why it is difficult to intubate a cat.

68. **The correct answer is 3.** An autoclave uses steam to sterilize instruments. Soap and water are used to clean the skin; disinfectants are used to clean surgical tables and instruments; and heat is used to make the steam used in an autoclave, so choices 1, 2, and 4 are incorrect.

69. **The correct answer is 4.** Nephrectomy is the name of the surgical procedure that removes a kidney. A lumpectomy is the procedure in which a lump is removed from breast tissue, so choice 1 is incorrect. Choices 2 and 3 are incorrect because

an appendectomy is the removal of the appendix, and a hysterectomy is the removal of the uterus.

70. **The correct answer is 1.** Adrenergic drugs are known as sympathomimetic agents because their pharmacologic effects often mimic behaviors of the sympathetic nervous system. Examples of adrenergic drugs include epinephrine and norepinephrine. Adrenergic drugs don't imitate the functions of the cardiovascular, skeletal, and lymphatic systems in choices 2, 3, and 4.

71. **The correct answer is 1.** Analgesics are given to animals prior to surgery for pain relief. Choices 2, 3, and 4 are incorrect because other anesthetic medications—not analgesics—are used for sedation, muscle relaxation, or anxiety.

72. **The correct answer is 4.** A scalpel is used to make cuts during surgery, and, therefore is not used to close incisions. Absorbable sutures (choice 1), tissue glue (choice 2), and staples (choice 3) are used to close incisions after surgery, so choices 1, 2, and 3 are incorrect.

73. **The correct answer is 1.** Gastric dilation-volvulus, also known as bloat, is a very serious and life-threatening condition in which the stomach fills up with air. It requires immediate surgery to correct. Choices 2, 3, and 4 are incorrect because these conditions do not require emergency surgery. A luxating patella is a condition in which a dog's kneecap slips out of place and causes pain. Hip dysplasia is a genetic disease of the hip joint in dogs. Ovariohysterectomy is the removal of reproductive organs in a female animal.

74. **The correct answer is 2.** Because rats lack emesis ability, they do not need to fast before surgery. Birds, cattle, and dogs should fast before surgery because they could regurgitate during the procedure, so choices 1, 3, and 4 are incorrect.

75. **The correct answer is 2.** Draping is the process of covering a patient and surrounding areas with a sterile cotton, paper, or plastic sheet prior to a surgical procedure. Choice 1 is incorrect because toweling means to gently wrap a bird or other small animal in a towel as a type of restraint. Disinfecting and sterilization (choices 3 and 4) are incorrect because they describe techniques used to clean and kill microorganisms on items.

76. **The correct answer is 1.** Either calculus or extraction forceps should be used to initially remove thick calculus from an animal's teeth during the dental prophylaxis. Choice 2 is incorrect because a scaler is used to remove any calculus that remains after the initial calculus removal. An irrigation needle is used to cleanse the area around a tooth and a periodontal probe is used to measure pocket depths around a tooth, so choices 3 and 4 are incorrect.

77. **The correct answer is 3.** Sutures over joints should be removed in two weeks, or 14 days. Choices 1 and 2 are incorrect because removing sutures over joints after 7 or 10 days is too early. Choice 4 is incorrect because waiting 21 days to remove the sutures is too long.

78. **The correct answer is 3.** A cystotomy is a surgical procedure in which an incision is made in the urinary bladder. This procedure is most commonly used to remove bladder stones. Choice 1 is incorrect because cystocentesis is a procedure in which a needle is inserted into the bladder to collect a urine sample. Choice 2 is incorrect because pyometra is an abnormality that afflicts the uterus of unspayed female animals. Choice 4 is incorrect because ovariohysterectomy is another name for the removal of reproductive organs in a female animal.

79. **The correct answer is 1.** Aspergillosis is a condition caused by a fungus that infects a bird's throat and lungs. It is usually caused by feeding a bird moldy bird seed. The best treatments for this condition are antibiotics and surgery to remove granulomas or lesions inside air sacs. Enteritis is a condition that affects a bird's intestines. Antibiotics are used to treat enteritis. Newcastle disease is a highly contagious disease that affects the respiratory system of birds kept in unsanitary conditions. This condition is not treatable. Hepatic lipidosis, or fatty liver disease, is a disease in which large amounts of fat are deposited in a bird's liver. A low-fat diet is the best course of treatment for hepatic lipidosis.

80. **The correct answer is 4.** The scaler and polisher use heat to clean, and they can harm the tooth pulp with heat if you use them for too long. Choices 1, 2, and 3 are incorrect because the scaler and the

polisher don't scratch the tooth enamel (choice 1), harm the gums (choice 2), or damage the root of the tooth (choice 3).

81. **The correct answer is 3.** Onchocerciasis is caused by a roundworm known as the *Onchocerca volvulus*. The female worm burrows in the horse's connective tissue and releases prelarvae into the horse's bloodstream causing an allergic reaction. This produces open sores usually found on the horse's neck, so choice 3 is correct. Choices 1, 2, and 4 are incorrect because onchocerciasis does not cause lameness, wheezing, or discolored feces. These may be signs of other serious conditions such as pinworms or Navicular disease.

82. **The correct answer is 2.** Buccal pad separators are used to hold back a guinea pig's cheeks during teeth examinations. Choice 1 is incorrect because hobbles are a type of bandage. Choice 3 is incorrect because a hemostat is a pair of grasping forceps used during surgical procedures. Choice 4 is incorrect because an ophthalmoscope is used to examine a patient's eyes.

83. **The correct answer is 3.** Used needles should always be placed in containers designated for sharp biomedical waste. Because a needle is considered biomedical waste, you should never flush it down the toilet or dispose of it in a trash receptacle, so choices 1 and 2 are incorrect. Choice 4 is incorrect because it is not safe to sterilize a needle for reuse.

84. **The correct answer is 4.** A root canal, dental prophylaxis, and extraction (choices 1, 2, and 3) are all common dental procedures for dogs. Choice 4 is correct because it is not a dental procedure. Periapical is the name for the tissue that surrounds the apex of tooth's root.

85. **The correct answer is 1.** Laboratory equipment should be sterilized in an autoclave, which uses heat and steam to sterilize equipment. Washing it in hot water (choice 2), submerging it in alcohol (choice 3), and scrubbing it with antibacterial soap (choice 4) are not so effective as autoclaving, so these choices are incorrect.

86. **The correct answer is 2.** Because rabbits have hypsodont teeth, they need a diet high in tough, fibrous plants to help keep their teeth worn down. When rabbits are not fed an adequate diet, their teeth are most likely to grow at an uneven rate and they could develop malocclusion, which is the misalignment of teeth. Choice 1 is incorrect because pulpitis is a condition that affects the pulp of the tooth. Choices 3 and 4 are incorrect because gingivitis and plaque are causes of periodontal disease.

87. **The correct answer is 1.** The condition in which a dog or cat is born with more teeth than usual is called supernumerary. Choice 2 is incorrect because oligodontia refers to being born with fewer teeth than normal. Choice 3 is incorrect because anodontia refers to being born with no teeth. Choice 4 is incorrect because deciduous refers to the first set of teeth, or primary set of teeth.

88. **The correct answer is 4.** Acepromazine is a tranquilizer that is used prior to anesthesia and surgery to sedate the animal and prevent vomiting. Choice 1 is incorrect because methocarbamol is a muscle relaxant. Choice 2 is incorrect because amoxicillin is an antibiotic used to treat bacterial infections. Choice 3 is incorrect because trifluridine is an antiviral ophthalmic drug.

89. **The correct answer is 3.** A young horse has 24 deciduous (also called temporary) teeth. An adult horse has between 36 and 44 permanent teeth. Choices 1 and 2 are incorrect because horses have more than 12 or 16 deciduous teeth. Choice 4 is incorrect because horses have fewer than 36 deciduous teeth.

90. **The correct answer is 2.** A Pasteur pipette, or an eyedropper, is a glass or plastic tube that has a rubber bulb at the top used to transfer small quantities of liquids. A Pasteur pipette would not be effective for disinfecting instruments, cleaning wounds, or picking up other instruments, so choices 1, 3, and 4 are incorrect.

91. **The correct answer is 1.** All used lab equipment and work surfaces should be cleaned daily. Larger pieces of equipment and work surfaces should be wiped down thoroughly using a rag or towel soaked with disinfectant. Smaller pieces of equipment, such as pipettes, should be soaked in a tub of disinfectant. Choices 2, 3, and 4 are incorrect because no more than a day should pass between laboratory cleanings.

92. The correct answer is 4. Fecal samples should be stored at cool temperatures and not at room temperature, so choice 4 is correct. Choices 1, 2, and 3 are incorrect because samples should be stored in an airtight container, and they can be contaminated by grass and soil.

93. The correct answer is 3. Smears should be dried by the air. Choices 1 and 2 are incorrect because a fan or a heater should not be used to dry a smear because they can damage the cells. Choice 4 is incorrect because blowing on the smear could contaminate the cells.

94. The correct answer is 4. Intravenous anesthesia is administered into a pig's auricular veins in its ear (choice 4). Intravenous anesthesia is not administered into a pig's hoof, neck, or snout (choices 1, 2, and 3).

95. The correct answer is 1. Chemicals, acids, and reagents should be stored in short clear and amber wide-based bottles with either a screw top or stopper. Choices 2, 3, and 4 are incorrect because chemicals, acids, and reagents should not be stored in thin, tall bottles, dark green bottles, or plastic bottles with snap-off caps.

96. The correct answer is 3. Cats are more prone to platelet clumping than horses, birds, and lizards; therefore, choices 1, 2, and 4 are incorrect.

97. The correct answer is 4. Basophilic cells pick up alkaline dyes and will turn blue or purple after staining. Basophilic cells don't turn red, orange, or green after staining, so choices 1, 2, and 3 are incorrect.

98. The correct answer is 2. Heparin is used to prevent blood from clotting. Choice 1 is incorrect because idoxuridine is a topical medication used to treat viral infections. Choice 3 is incorrect because enalapril is used to treat heart and vascular conditions. Choice 4 is incorrect because praziquantel is a parasite-control drug used to treat animals with tapeworms.

99. The correct answer is 2. Lens paper should be used to clean the lenses of a microscope to avoid scratching the lenses. Disinfectant solutions, soap and water, and an autoclave are used to clean and sterilize other parts of the microscope, so choices 1, 3, and 4 are incorrect.

100. The correct answer is 1. A rabbit's ears are generally the best places to collect blood samples. The veins running through rabbits' ears make them the best place from which to collect blood samples. Choice 2 is incorrect because some reptiles, not rabbits, have blood samples taken from their tails. Choice 3 is incorrect because blood samples are not normally taken from a rabbit's feet. The jugular vein, located in the neck, is a popular blood collection location for species such as dogs and cats, but not for rabbits, so choice 4 is incorrect.

101. The correct answer is 1. When giving a dog an injection in the external jugular vein, it is important to avoid the carotid artery, which lies parallel to the vein. Choices 2, 3, and 4 are incorrect because the cephalic vein, femoral artery, and saphenous vein are located in a dog's legs, not in the neck.

102. The correct answer is 2. A fecal specimen bottle should be labeled on its sides because if you remove the labeled lid, the specimen is no longer labeled. All specimens should be properly labeled at all times. Choice 1 is incorrect because labels are not more easily removed from the lid than from the bottle. Choice 3 is incorrect because labeling methods are concerned with safety and accuracy more than with professionalism. Choice 4 is incorrect because fecal specimens need lids.

103. The correct answer is 4. Crenation is a condition that causes red blood cells to shrink and form notches around their edges. Crenation does not cause cells to divide, mutate, or expand, so choices 1, 2, and 3 are incorrect.

104. The correct answer is 1. To screen for carbon monoxide poisoning, you should collect a sample of whole blood. Choices 2, 3, and 4 are incorrect because urine, serum, and stomach contents are not so effective as whole blood in determining carbon monoxide poisoning.

105. The correct answer is 2. Anuria is a serious condition in which the kidneys fail to excrete urine. Choice 1 is incorrect because pyometra is an abnormality that afflicts the uterus of unspayed female animals. Hematuria is the presence of blood in urine, so choice 3 is incorrect. Choice 4 is incorrect because polydipsia is a condition that causes excessive thirst.

106. The correct answer is 4. Exposing the sample to full sunlight is most likely to damage a whole blood sample because the sunlight can cause red blood cells to rupture. Choice 1 is incorrect because storing the sample in a cold area (in temperatures above freezing) can help preserve the sample. Choice 2 is incorrect because inverting or rolling the sample tube will not damage the sample. Shaking the tube can damage it. Choice 3 is incorrect because using a wide-gauge needle is preferred to using a smaller-gauge needle, which could cause red blood cells to rupture.

107. The correct answer is 4. A female adult golden retriever should weigh 60–70 pounds. Choices 1 and 2 are incorrect because these weight ranges are too low. Choice 4 is incorrect because this weight range is too high.

108. The correct answer is 2. The best urine collection container is an opaque plastic container with a screw-on lid. The opaque plastic container keeps the sample from being exposed to light and the screw-on lid ensures the sample does not leak during transport. Choices 1, 3, and 4 are incorrect because a clear plastic container could expose the sample to too much light and a snap-on lid could allow the sample to leak from its container.

109. The correct answer is 3. A ferret usually lives for an average of 5–7 years. Choices 1 and 2 are incorrect because these age ranges are too low. Choice 4 is incorrect because this age range is too high.

110. The correct answer is 1. Rabies is a virus that affects the central nervous system of animals. It's transmitted in the saliva of infected animals. Rabies is not spread through blood, urine, or feces, so choices 2, 3, and 4 are incorrect.

111. The correct answer is 1. The best time to collect a voided urine sample is right after the patient wakes up. This is the best time to collect a urine sample because the patient's bladder has filled with urine for 6–8 hours, and it will give the most accurate results. Choices 2, 3, and 4 are incorrect because urine samples taken throughout the day are less reliable due to fluctuations from eating, drinking, and activity.

112. The correct answer is 2. Colitis is the inflammation of the large colon. It causes symptoms such as diarrhea, abdominal cramps, gas, and bloating. Because colitis affects the large colon, it does not affect an animal's ability to produce urine or regurgitate, so choices 1 and 4 are incorrect. Choice 3 is incorrect because constipation is not a symptom of colitis.

113. The correct answer is 1. Blood culture tubes should be collected before any other samples because they must be sterile for accurate results. Choice 2, 3, and 4 are incorrect because these samples should be taken after blood culture tubes.

114. The correct answer is 2. Coprophagia is the practice of eating feces. This is a normal behavior for dogs and is caused by a variety of reasons, including boredom and hunger. Choices 1, 3, and 4 are incorrect because coprophagia is not the practice of eating rocks, grass, or trash.

115. The correct answer is 1. Unconsciousness and hemorrhaging are life-threatening conditions that require immediate medical care. Choices 2, 3, and 4 are incorrect because this example is a life-threatening emergency. Gaping wounds and dislocated bones or joints are examples of serious emergencies. Minor burns and wounds are examples of minor emergencies. A nonemergency is any type of injury that doesn't require medical attention.

116. The correct answer is 2. A laceration is an irregular-shaped open wound with jagged, uneven edges. An abrasion is an open wound that only affects the top layers of the skin, so choice 1 is incorrect. Choice 3 is incorrect because a puncture is a deep open wound with a small entrance site to the wound. Choice 4 is incorrect because a contusion, or a bruise, is a closed wound in which capillaries under the skin break and cause swelling and discoloration.

117. The correct answer is 1. During plane 1, which is considered light anesthesia, the animal has the ability to blink and swallow. Choices 2, 3, and 4 are incorrect because the animal loses the ability to blink during these planes.

118. The correct answer is 1. When you ship whole blood to a lab, you must not allow the whole blood specimens to directly touch ice because some of the cells in the specimens could be destroyed. Choices 2 and 4 are incorrect because direct contact with ice packs could harm the whole blood. Choice 3 is incorrect because whole blood must be kept cold while it is shipped to a lab.

119. **The correct answer is 4.** Scissors, not forceps, are generally used to cut through sutures, so choice 4 is correct. Forceps are used to grasp and hold tissue during surgery, to pick up sterile surgical instruments during preparation for surgery, and to remove calculus from an animal's teeth during dental prophylaxis, so choices 1, 2, and 3 are incorrect.

120. **The correct answer is 1.** Universities are not permitted to mail pathological specimens unless they have special permission from the post office. Dental practices, veterinary practices, and laboratories (choices 2, 3, and 4) are permitted to mail pathological specimens.

121. **The correct answer is 1.** When you occlude, or block, the proximal part of the vein, the vein is easier to see and identify. Choice 2 is incorrect because occluding the vein does not make the area numb. Choice 3 is incorrect because patients do not become relaxed by occluding their veins. Choice 4 is incorrect because occlusion of the proximal part of the vein before taking the sample does not stop excessive bleeding.

122. **The correct answer is 2.** A Jackson catheter is designed to be used on cats. The Tieman's catheter (choice 1) is incorrect because it is a soft and flexible catheter used for female dogs. A Foley catheter is a flexible catheter with a balloon at the tip and mostly used for female dogs, so choice 3 is incorrect. A Robinson catheter (choice 4) is not correct because it is a flexible catheter used for short-term drainage of urine.

123. **The correct answer is 2.** Snakes do not have a urinary bladder. Since cats, ferrets, and cattle have urinary bladders, choices 1, 3, and 4 are incorrect.

124. **The correct answer is 2.** Imidacloprid, also known as Advantage®, is a topical medication that is applied directly to the skin to prevent parasites such as fleas. Lincomycin is an oral antibiotic used to treat bacterial infections, so choice 1 is

incorrect. Choice 3 is incorrect because xylazine is a sedative and muscle relaxant given orally or by injection. Nitroprusside is a muscle relaxant given intravenously, so choice 4 is incorrect.

125. **The correct answer is 3.** Cotton swabs are the best instruments to collect cells from the ear canal. Collecting cells from the sensitive ear canal does not require sharp instruments such as needles and scalpels, so choices 1 and 2 are incorrect. Choice 4, forceps, is incorrect because forceps would not properly collect the skin cells.

126. **The correct answer is 4.** Chestnuts are nontoxic to dogs. Choices 1, 2, and 3 are incorrect because antifreeze, cocoa mulch, and azaleas (a type of plant) are toxic to dogs if they are ingested.

127. **The correct answer is 2.** Dry gums are a symptom of dehydration. Dry eyes, dry hair, and dry skin are not generally indicators of dehydration, so choices 1, 3, and 4 are incorrect.

128. **The correct answer is 4.** A cat is an example of an animal with brachydont teeth. Brachydont teeth have short crowns and well-developed roots. Choices 1, 2, and 3 are incorrect because a rabbit, horse, and deer are all examples of animals with hypsodont teeth. Hypsodont teeth have high or deep crowns and short roots.

129. **The correct answer is 3.** The number of canine blood groups is 8. These groups are: DEA 1.1, DEA 1.2, DEA 3, DEA 4, DEA 5, DEA 6, DEA 7, and DEA 8. Choices 1 and 2 are incorrect because these choices indicate too few canine blood groups. Choice 4 is incorrect because this choice indicates too many canine blood groups.

130. **The correct answer is 4.** Infection is a common cause of high body temperature, so choice 4 is correct. Choices 1, 2, and 3 are incorrect because general anesthesia, shock, and circulatory collapse are all common causes of low body temperature.

131. **The correct answer is 3.** Unconscious animals shouldn't be treated with emetics, so choice 3 is correct. Animals that are seizing, lethargic, or unconscious should not be treated with emetics. Choice 1 is incorrect because, in some cases of poisoning, dogs should be treated with emetics. Choice 2 is incorrect because animals that are having seizures shouldn't be given emetics. Choice

4 is not correct because dogs that eat toxic plants can sometimes receive emetics.

132. The correct answer is 2. The veterinarian used delayed primary closure on the patient. This delayed closure is used when the wound is contaminated and could get infected if it is closed immediately. Choice 1 is incorrect because primary closure is when a wound is cleaned and closed immediately. Choice 3 is incorrect because tertiary closure is not a real type of closure. Secondary closure, choice 4, is incorrect because this type of closure occurs after five days.

133. The correct answer is 3. You should avoid tending to the infected patient before other patients. You should care for the infected patient after other patients so that you don't spread the infection to other animals. Choice 1 is incorrect because you should put the patient's chart outside its room so that others can read the chart without going into the patient's room. Choice 2 is not correct because you should always wear disposable protective clothing when you're working with an infected animal. Choice 4 is incorrect because you should always dispose of used needles in the biomedical waste.

134. The correct answer is 1. The placement of sutures too close to wound edges is a common reason that wounds don't heal, so choice 1 is correct. Increased circulation helps wounds heal, so choice 2 is incorrect. Absorbable sutures being left on a wound for an extended period of time is not a common reason for a nonhealing wound because absorbable sutures generally stay on the body until the body absorbs them. Therefore, choice 3 is incorrect. Too much moisture accumulation prevents wounds from healing, and too little moisture at the wound is not a reason for a wound not to heal, so choice 4 is not correct.

135. The correct answer is 1. The veterinarian's note means the patient should get the drug by mouth three times per day. The abbreviation *PO* means "by mouth," and the abbreviation *t.i.d.* means "three times per day." Choices 2, 3, and 4 are incorrect because "intravenously" is abbreviated using *IV*, and "four times per day" is abbreviated using *q.i.d.*

136. The correct answer is 4. A puncture wound would most likely be caused by contact with a fish hook. Puncture wounds are wounds that do not show obvious signs of trauma on the skin, but go deep into the tissue. Choice 1 is incorrect because excessive head shaking often leads to hematomas. Choice 2 is not correct because exposure to broken glass would likely cause an incision wound. A road or traffic accident could cause wounds such as lacerations, shears, and contusions, so choice 3 is not correct.

137. The correct answer is 3. Interphase is not a stage of mitosis, so choice 3 is correct. The four stages of mitosis are anaphase, metaphase, prophase, and telophase. Mitosis is the process of cell division that takes place in the nucleus of a dividing cell. It results in two daughter nuclei that have the same number of chromosomes as the parent nucleus. Interphase refers to all stages of the cell cycle other than mitosis.

138. The correct answer is 2. Histology is a branch of anatomy that deals with the tissues of the body. Anatomy is the study of the body as a whole, so choice 1 is incorrect. Physiology, choice 3, is incorrect because it is a branch of biology that deals with the physical and chemical processes of living organisms. Choice 4 is incorrect because pathology is the study of disease.

139. The correct answer is 1. A CAT scan (computed tomography or CT scan) uses X-rays to scan the body for brain and spinal cord disorders. An endoscopy is used to explore the digestive system, so choice 2 is incorrect. An ultrasound produces an image of an internal organ, muscle, or tendon, so choice 3 is incorrect. Choice 4 is incorrect because a rhinoscopy examines the nasal cavity and nasopharynx (back of the throat).

140. The correct answer is 3. A scalpel is used to makes cuts in the skin. Scissors are used to cut through sutures. Needle holders are used to close up wounds. Forceps are used to grasp and hold tissues. Therefore, choices 1, 2, and 4 are incorrect.

141. The correct answer is 2. Most oxygen tanks are usually colored green so they can be easily recognized. Choices 1, 3, and 4 are incorrect because generally these are not colors of oxygen tanks.

142. The correct answer is 4. An ophthalmoscope is an instrument used to examine the eyes. Choices 1, 2, and 3 are incorrect because this instrument is not used to examine the ears, mouth, or heart of a patient.

143. The correct answer is 1. Since the instrument hit the floor, it is no longer sterile, and you should replace it with a sterile instrument. You should never place a contaminated instrument with sterile instruments, so choice 2 is incorrect. Choices 3 and 4 are incorrect because washing the instrument or soaking it in alcohol takes too much time and does not even sterilize the instrument.

144. The correct answer is 2. Surgical removal of the lens of the affected eye or eyes is the best course of treatment for cataracts in animals. Choice 1 is incorrect because this is a course of treatment for conjunctivitis. Medicated eye drops will not treat the cataracts, so choice 3 is not correct. Choice 4 is incorrect because the surgical removal of the eye or eyes is unwarranted for cataracts.

145. The correct answer is 1. The veterinarian's order means you should give the animal nothing to eat or drink. The abbreviation NPO, which stands for the Latin "nil per os," means nothing by mouth and indicates that the animal should not be given anything by mouth, including food and water. Choices 2, 3, and 4 are incorrect because the animal should not have any amount of food or water.

146. The correct answer is 1. Mineralized components of bone are the only pieces of the skeletal system that can be seen clearly in radiographs. Lesions in bones may appear on certain films, but they are oftentimes difficult to detect. Articular cartilage and the osteoid matrix are soft tissues that won't show up on plain radiographs. Therefore, choices 2, 3, and 4 are incorrect.

147. The correct answer is 1. A contusion, which is a bruise, is a closed wound in which capillaries under the skin break and cause swelling and discoloration. It does not usually require bandaging. A laceration is an irregular-shaped open wound with jagged, uneven edges. An abrasion is an open wound that only affects the top layers of the skin. Choice 3 is incorrect because a puncture is a deep open wound with a small entrance site to the wound. These wounds usually need bandaging, so choices 2, 3, and 4 are incorrect.

148. The correct answer is 3. When you clean a patient's kennel, you should rinse detergent and disinfectant thoroughly so the animal does not have an adverse reaction to the detergent or disinfectant. Choice 1 is incorrect because you should not put the patient in with another animal. Choice 2 is incorrect because you should take out everything, including food bowls, from the kennel before you clean it. Choice 4 is incorrect because you should thoroughly dry the kennel and not leave it to air dry.

149. The correct answer is 2. When a material such as a radioactive dye is administered intravenously, it is injected into the bloodstream through the veins, which are large blood vessels that carry blood toward the heart. Choices 1, 3, and 4 are incorrect because drugs that are administered intravenously are not injected into the arteries, capillaries, or arterioles.

150. The correct answer is 2. The disinfectant triclosan would most likely be used on the skin. Triclosan is a mild disinfectant that does not usually irritate tissue. Bleach (choice 1), formaldehyde (choice 3), and ammonia (choice 4) are not correct because these disinfectants can irritate the skin and can be toxic to animals and humans.

151. The correct answer is 4. The surgical scrub should include your hands and forearms. Washing the hands, wrists, and forearms is an important aseptic technique that will help decrease the likelihood of infection. Choice 1 is incorrect because the scrub should be completed with water that is warm, but a comfortable temperature. Choice 2 is incorrect because the surgical scrub should last longer than 60 seconds. Choice 3 is not correct because all jewelry and watches should be taken off before you perform the surgical scrub.

152. The correct answer is 3. Not documenting a minor chemical spill in the accident book is an example of an unethical act. All chemical spills, regardless of how minor they are, should be recorded. Choices 1 and 2 are incorrect because these are examples of ethical procedures. Choice 4 is incorrect because forgetting to do something is not an unethical act.

153. The correct answer is 1. Before giving the patient intravenous fluids with a catheter, you should first clip the patient's fur. The patient's skin should be clean before you give it a catheter to avoid infection. By clipping the fur, you make the area easier to clean and the vein easier to see. Choices 2, 3, and 4 are incorrect because you tape the catheter to the patient's body (choice 2), disinfect the skin (choice 3), and occlude the vein (choice 4) after you clip the fur.

154. The correct answer is 2. A nuclear scintigraphy is a nuclear test used to scan a horse's bones. First, the animal is injected with a radioactive dye that accumulates around inflamed bones. Then, the horse is scanned with a gamma camera to examine the function of its bones. Nuclear scintigraphy is not used to examine a horse's muscles (choice 1), ears (choice 3), or eyes (choice 4), so those are incorrect.

155. The correct answer is 1. Radiation is used to shrink or destroy tumors. It uses photons, electrons, or gamma rays to destroy the nucleus of the cell in a tumor. It is not used to treat bronchitis, which is the inflammation of the air passages of the lungs, so choice 2 is incorrect. Choice 3 is incorrect because radiation is not used to treat osteoarthritis, which is a type of arthritis or degenerative joint disease. Radiation is not used to treat a urinary tract infection, so choice 4 is incorrect.

156. The correct answer is 2. The endotracheal tube is placed in the animal's windpipe to carry oxygen and gases to the animal's lungs. Choice 1 is incorrect because this is a function of the inhalation hose. Choice 3 is incorrect because this is a function of the exhalation hose. Choice 4 is incorrect because this is a function of the exhalation valve.

157. The correct answer is 1. During a renal scintigraphy, the animal is injected with a radioactive dye and then is scanned with a gamma camera to examine the function of its kidneys. Choice 2 is incorrect because an ultrasound is a test that produces an image of an internal organ, muscle, or tendon. Choice 3 is incorrect because cystocentesis is a procedure in which a needle is inserted into the bladder to collect a urine sample. Choice 4 is incorrect because a urine analysis is a test that examines the patient's urine.

158. The correct answer is 3. Portal scintigraphy is a nuclear test that is used to diagnoses portosystemic shunts in dogs and cats. The portal system is made up of blood vessels that collect blood from the stomach and intestines and then sends the blood to the liver before it goes to the heart. A portosystemic shunt causes the blood to bypass the liver before it goes to the heart and causes toxins to build up in the body. During a portal scintigraphy, radioactive dye is injected into the animal's intestines and then the animal is scanned with a gamma camera to examine the tract of the radioactive dye. Choices 1, 2, and 4 are incorrect because these nuclear tests examine the kidneys, thyroid, and brain.

159. The correct answer is 2. While a PET scan, CAT scan, and MRI can be helpful when diagnosing bone problems, an X-ray should be the first test performed prior to a bone scintigraphy, which is a nuclear test used to examine the bones. An X-ray can determine if pain is caused by something minor, such as a fracture or sprain. A bone scintigraphy is used to diagnose more advanced bone problems.

160. The correct answer is 3. Local anesthetics help diagnose lameness in horses. Choices 1, 2, and 3 are incorrect because local anesthetics don't typically help diagnose lameness in pigs, cattle, or sheep.

161. The correct answer is 3. MRIs do not affect pregnant animals, so a 9-month-old pregnant ferret with a cloth bandage would be an ideal candidate for an MRI. Because an MRI uses a magnetic field, animals that have pacemakers, microchips, or other metal objects embedded in their bodies should not have a MRI, so choices 1, 2, and 4 are incorrect.

162. The correct answer is 3. Choice 3 is false because a rebreathing anesthesia machine is used on animals weighing more than 10 pounds. Choices 1, 2, and 4 are accurate statements regarding rebreathing anesthesia machines.

163. The correct answer is 1. An ultrasound is helpful in confirming if an animal is pregnant. Choices 2, 3, and 4 are incorrect because an X-ray would be used to diagnose a luxating patella, a bone fracture, or hip dysplasia, all of which affect bones and are easily diagnosed with an X-ray.

164. The correct answer is 1. After the animal receives medication to help it relax, it is put in an unconscious state either by an injectable anesthetic or an inhalant anesthesia. Choices 2 and 3 are incorrect because surgery is performed on the animal, and the animal is monitored until it wakes during the third stage of anesthesia. Choice 4 is incorrect because the animal is given medications to relax it before it is placed in an unconscious state.

165. **The correct answer is 3.** Bamboo is nontoxic to a cat. Choices 1, 2, and 4 are incorrect because alfalfa, baby's breath, and juniper are poisonous to cats.

166. **The correct answer is 4.** Shivering, vomiting, and urination are normal side effects of anesthesia, but dehydration is not a normal side effect. Therefore, choices 1, 2, and 3 are incorrect.

167. **The correct answer is 3.** During planes 3 and 4 of the third stage of anesthesia, breathing becomes difficult for the patient because the patient begins to lose the use of their chest and abdominal muscles, so assisted ventilation should be used during this time. Choices 1, 2, and 4 are incorrect because the patient is able to breathe on his or her own during these planes.

168. **The correct answer is 1.** Animals that have collapsed, especially those with injuries to the abdomen or back, should be moved only with a stretcher. Therefore, a dog that has collapsed with abdominal injuries should be moved with a stretcher. Choices 2, 3, and 4 are incorrect because these animals can be moved without the help of a stretcher.

169. **The correct answer is 4.** To test capillary refill time, press on the patient's limb. The color should change from pink to white and return to pink again within 2 seconds. If it takes longer for the color to return, then this is an indication that the capillaries are compromised and the anesthesia is too deep. Choices 1, 2, and 3 are incorrect because these are not effective ways to test capillary refill time.

170. **The correct answer is 1.** As part of the preanesthetic screening process, a thorough examination is performed along with blood tests and an electrocardiogram (EKG) to check for any abnormalities. Choices 2, 3, and 4 are incorrect because these choices refer to steps that are taken prior to surgery.

171. **The correct answer is 3.** The rotating turret is part of the nosepiece, which holds the objective lenses. Choice 1 is incorrect because the stage holds the slides on a microscope and is located above the substage condenser. Choice 2 is incorrect because a rheostat controls the intensity of the light and is located in the base of the microscope. Choice 4 is incorrect because the optical tube is housed within the body of the tube.

172. **The correct answer is 4.** A patient's heart rate and rhythm can be monitored during anesthesia by using a stethoscope to listen to the chest, placing a hand directly on the chest to feel for heart rhythms, or using an electrocardiogram to record the electrical activity of the heart. A ventilator is used to move air in and out of the lungs of a patient that cannot breathe on its own and is not used to monitor the patient's heart rate and rhythm during anesthesia.

173. **The correct answer is 3.** Because a Persian cat is brachycephalic, it can be more difficult to place an endotracheal tube. Animals that are brachycephalic have shortened faces and noses that make their faces appear "pushed in." Choices 1, 2, and 4 are incorrect because Akita dogs, Siamese cats, and German shepherd dogs are not types of brachycephalic animals.

174. **The correct answer is 4.** ADME stands for the four key physiological processes that determine the course of a drug in the body: absorption, distribution, metabolism, and elimination. Atrophy, diet medicine, and excretion are not any of the four key physiological processes, so choices 1, 2, and 3 are incorrect.

175. **The correct answer is 3.** Obesity affects a dog's heart and lungs and could cause cardiac arrest when the dog is put under anesthesia. Anesthetics are absorbed into a dog's fat, so an overweight dog will spend more time under anesthesia. Anesthetics are broken down by the liver and a fatty liver is not so effective at breaking down anesthetics as a normal liver. Anesthesia does not affect the bladder in overweight dogs, so choice 3 is correct.

176. **The correct answer is 4.** The Macintosh is a curved laryngoscope blade. The Miller, Wisconsin, and

Phillips are types of straight laryngoscope blades, so choices 1, 2, and 3 are incorrect.

177. **The correct answer is 3.** When performing an endotracheal intubation on a dog, you should first pull out the tongue to get a clear view of the animal's throat. Checking for air leakage, inserting the tube, and tying the tube in place are all steps that follow pulling out the tongue, so choices 1, 2, and 4 are incorrect.

178. **The correct answer is 2.** Wet or soiled bandages should be removed and replaced with dry bandages, so choice 2 is correct. Choice 1 is incorrect because bandages on patients' limbs should cover the entire limb so swelling doesn't occur. Choice 3 is not correct because a bandage is too tight if you cannot put your finger between the skin and the bandage. Choice 4 is incorrect because pressure bandages should be replaced every 12, not 24, hours.

179. **The correct answer is 3.** After the endotracheal tube is placed, the cuff should be inflated to form a tight seal. Choice 1 is incorrect because the cuff should be deflated after removing the endotracheal tube. Choice 2 is incorrect because the patient should be moved into position after the cuff is inflated. Choice 4 is incorrect because the patient should be anesthetized before the endotracheal tube is placed.

180. **The correct answer is 1.** Scored tablets are the only tablets that should be divided because they are guaranteed by the manufacturer to have equal amounts of the drug distributed throughout the tablet. Choices 2 and 4 are incorrect because soft and hard gelatin tablets contain medication in either liquid or powder form that is surrounded by a hard or soft gelatin layer that dissolves in the stomach. Layered tablets contain layers of medication that are covered by other layers to delay the release of the medication, so choice 3 is incorrect.

181. **The correct answer is 2.** A non-rebreathing anesthesia machine does not contain an oxygen flush valve. A non-rebreathing anesthesia machine does contain an endotracheal tube, a pressure reducing valve, and a flowmeter, so choices 1, 3, and 4 are incorrect.

182. **The correct answer is 1.** Monophyodont animals develop only one set of teeth in their lifetimes.

Choice 2 is incorrect because animals with hypsodont teeth have high or deep crowns and short roots. Choice 3 is incorrect because diphyodont animals develop two sets of teeth (deciduous and permanent) in their lifetimes. Choice 4 is incorrect because animals with brachydont teeth have short crowns and well-developed roots.

183. **The correct answer is 4.** Drugs administered to meat and dairy animals will be in the meat and dairy products. Special consideration must be made when choosing types and amounts of drugs for these animals because their meat and milk could be contaminated by the drugs. Choice 1 is incorrect because dosing varies for all different animal species and sizes. Choice 2 is incorrect because the owners of bovines, pigs, and goats are just as likely to want their animals operated on as other animal owners. Choice 3 is incorrect because bovines, pigs, and goats all react differently to anesthesia, and they (as a group) are not more sensitive to the drugs than other animals.

184. **The correct answer is 2.** Aminoglycosides are used as antibiotics and are derived from bacteria of the *Streptomyces* genus. *Borrelia* and *Leptospira* are both genera of bacteria from the Spirochete phylum. *Thermotoga* is a genus of bacteria from the Thermotogae phylum.

185. **The correct answer is 4.** Exercise does not help prevent periodontal disease in dogs. Choices 1, 2, and 3 are incorrect because daily tooth brushing (choice 1), diet (choice 2), and chewing on bones (choice 3) help prevent periodontal disease in dogs.

186. **The correct answer is 3.** Atropine is given to a patient before anesthesia to help control the heart rate and the amount of saliva produced. Choice 1 is incorrect because griseofulvin is an antifungal drug. Choice 2 is incorrect because diazepam is a tranquilizer. Choice 4 is incorrect because erythromycin inhibits bacteria growth.

187. **The correct answer is 1.** When you shine a light into the patient's eye, you can test the pupillary reflex during anesthesia. The pupil constricts at the beginning of the third stage of anesthesia and does nothing by the middle of the third stage of anesthesia. Choice 2 is incorrect because touching the corner of the patient's eye tests the palpebral reflex. Choice 3 is incorrect because pulling on the

patient's limbs tests the withdrawal reflex. Choice 4 is incorrect because stimulating the larynx tests the laryngeal reflex.

188. **The correct answer is 4.** Styptic powder is used to contract the blood vessels and clot bleeding in cats, dogs, and birds, especially when the animal's nail is clipped too close to the nail bed. Choices 1, 2, and 3 are incorrect because these treatments are not used to control bleeding. Ketamine is a rapidly acting general anesthetic. Meperidine is a sedative used to alleviate pain. St. John's Wort is an herbal remedy used to treat a variety of symptoms including anxiety, upset stomach, and insomnia.

189. **The correct answer is 2. The surgery table should be disinfected before adjusting the table, placing a heating blanket on it, and performing the draping process, so choices 1, 3, and 4 are incorrect.**

190. **The correct answer is 4.** When anesthesia is administered intravenously it has the fastest effect. Anesthesia that is administered intravenously takes effect almost immediately. Choices 1 and 2 are incorrect because anesthesia administered subcutaneously or intramuscularly takes 10–15 minutes to begin working. Choice 3 is incorrect because anesthesia that is administered transdermally could take a few hours to begin working effectively.

191. **The correct answer is 2.** Prehensile organs are those that allow animals to grasp food and pull it into their mouths to eat. Choice 1 is incorrect because the lingual surface is the part of the teeth in an animal's mouth that faces the tongue. Choice 3 is incorrect because it is also referring to teeth, not lips. The teeth in an upper arcade are those in the upper part of an animal's mouth. Longitudinal muscles, choice 4, are found in the gut and are unrelated to a horse's lips.

192. **The correct answer is 3.** A splint is applied to fractures and dislocations of bones, not closed wounds. Pain medication, bandages, and cold compresses are all treatments for closed wounds, so choices 1, 2, and 4 are correct.

193. **The correct answer is 2.** A PET (positron emission tomography) scan is a nuclear test used to evaluate the function of the organs and tissues within the body. During a PET scan, a radioactive material is injected into the body and is traced using a gamma camera. A computer produces images of the organs through which the radioactive material flows. Choice 1 is incorrect because a CAT scan uses X-rays to scan the body for brain and spinal cord disorders. An MRI uses a magnetic field to produce images of the inside of the body, so choice 3 is incorrect. Choice 4 is incorrect because myelography is the radiographic examination of the spinal cord.

194. **The correct answer is 1.** Choices 2, 3, and 4 are incorrect because lidocaine is an example of a local anesthetic. A local anesthetic is given before surgery to provide pain control for a specific area of the body.

195. **The correct answer is 1.** The parvovirus is a life-threatening virus that can be passed to a dog through contact with infected fecal matter. It can also be transmitted by insects or rodents that come into contact with infected fecal matter. It is unlikely to be spread by contaminated water, sick humans, or spoiled food, so choices 2, 3, and 4 are incorrect.

196. **The correct answer is 1.** A lavender Vacutainer with a pink collecting pot indicates a sample of whole blood and the anticoagulant EDTA (ethylenediaminetetraacetic acid). A green or green and orange Vacutainer with an orange collecting pot indicates an anticoagulant of heparin, so choice 2 is incorrect. Choice 3 is incorrect because sodium citrate is found in a light blue Vacutainer. Oxalate fluoride is found in a gray Vacutainer with a yellow collecting pot, so choice 4 is incorrect.

197. **The correct answer is 2.** The main purpose of the anesthesia machine is to deliver a mixture of oxygen and anesthetic gas to the animal during surgery. Choices 1, 3, and 4 are incorrect because these are not functions of the anesthesia machine.

198. **The correct answer is 2.** Animals are highly susceptible to hypothermia, so a heating pad should be placed under the patient during surgery. Choices 1, 3, and 4 are incorrect reasons to use a heating pad during surgery.

199. **The correct answer is 3.** Ketamine is a type of general anesthetic that is used to block pain sensation and prevent movement during surgery.

Choices 1 and 4 are incorrect because diazepam and midazolam are sedatives used to relax animals before surgery. Choice 2 is incorrect because bupivacaine is a local anesthetic for pain control.

200. **The correct answer is 2.** Use the formula Dose = body weight × dosage / concentration of drug. To get the percentage solution into mg/ml, multiply by 10. Dose = 13.6 kg × 10 mg/kg / 2.0% × 10 mg/ml = 136 mg / 20 mg/ml, so choice 2, 6.8 ml. is correct. Choice 1 is incorrect because that dose is too low. Choices 3 and 4 are incorrect because those doses are too high.

APPENDIXES

Medical Terms Used on the VTNE

The VTNE contains a number of medical terms and abbreviations that may be unfamiliar to you. Review these common medical terms and abbreviations and their definitions so you can recognize them on the VTNE.

Abduction—The movement of a limb away from the body

Ad lib—As much as desired

A.D.—Right ear

Addison's disease—A disease in which the adrenal gland produces an insufficient amount of hormones

Adduction—The movement of a limb toward the body

Adrenal gland—One of a pair of endocrine glands that produces hormones such as cortisol and epinephrine

ALT—Alanine aminotransferase

Analgesia—Decreased pain sensibilities

Anatomy—A subbranch of biology that deals with the structure of living things

Anesthesia—Loss of pain sensation

Anterior—Located toward the front of the body

Antiseptic—A substance that inhibits the growth of bacteria

Anuria—A condition in which no urine is produced

A.S.—Left ear

AST—Aspartate aminotransferase

A.U.—Both ears

Benign—Mild or not life threatening

b.i.d.—An abbreviation meaning *two times per day* (every 12 hours)

Bilateral—Located on both sides of the body

Biopsy—Removal of tissues from the body for examination

Bone marrow—A soft tissue made up of blood vessels and connective tissues found in bones

Brachycephalic—The state of being short-faced or broad-headed

BUN—Blood urea nitrogen

Carapace—The upper shell of a turtle, tortoise, or crab

Carcinogen—A substance that causes cancer

Castration—Sterilization of a male animal

Cataracts—Loss of transparency of the lens of the eye

CK—Creatinine kinase

CNS—Central nervous system

Coagulation—The chemical reaction that thickens liquid blood into a clot

Colitis—An inflammation or infection of the colon

Congenital—Present at birth; acquired during pre-natal development

Conjunctivitis—An inflammation of the conjunctiva, or the lining of the eyelid and the front of the eyeball

CRT—Capillary refill time

Cushing's disease—A disease in which the adrenal gland produces an abnormally large amount of hormones

Cytology—A branch of biology that focuses on the structures and functions of cells

Dermatitis—The inflammation of the skin

Disinfection—The use of chemicals or heat to kill germs

Distal—Located away from the body

Distemper—A viral disease that causes a severe and often fatal systemic illness in dogs

Diuresis—An increase in urine production

Diurnal—Of or relating to the daytime

Dorsal—Toward the back of the body

Ecdysis—The process in which reptiles shed the external layers of the skin

ECG—Electrocardiogram

Ectoparasite—A parasite that lives on the outside surface or skin of another animal

Edema—A condition that causes the tissues of the body to retain too much fluid

EDTA—Anticoagulant ethylenediaminete traacetic acid

Elizabethan Collar—A plastic cone-shaped collar used on animals to prevent licking or biting of the skin

Emaciation—The severe loss of body weight

Endotracheal tube—A tube placed into the animal's trachea (windpipe) to allow oxygen and gases to be breathed into the lungs

Estrus—The time when a female animal is fertile

Euthanasia—The act of killing an animal humanely because it is severely injured or helplessly ill

Feces—Wastes excreted through the anus from the large intestine

FeLV—Feline leukemia virus

FFD—Film focal distance

FIP—Feline infectious peritonitis

FIV—Feline immunodeficiency virus

Fluoroscopy—An X-ray procedure in which X-rays are transmitted through the body onto a fluorescent screen

Fracture—The breaking of bone

Gastric dilatation-volvulus (bloat)—A condition caused by expanding gas in which the stomach distends or becomes enlarged, which includes a complete rotation of the stomach that prevents gas from escaping

Gastritis—Inflammation of the stomach

GI—Gastrointestinal

Gingivitis— Inflammation of the gums

HCT—Hematocrit

Heartworm—A parasitic worm that lives and reproduces in the chambers of an animal's heart

Hematology—A branch of science that studies blood.

Hematoma—A mass of blood within the tissue

Hematuria—The presence of blood in urine

Hemostat—A surgical instrument used to clamp blood vessels

Hip dysplasia—Developmental, orthopedic condition that causes abnormal formation of the hip joint socket and leads to joint damage

Hot spot—Inflammation of the skin frequently caused by flea bites, allergies, or bacteria

Hyperglycemia—Higher than normal levels of glucose in the blood

Hyperthermia—Increased body temperature

Hypothermia—Decreased body temperature

ID—Intradermal

IM—Intramuscular

Immunity—A condition in which the animal's immune system is able to protect the body from a disease-causing agent

Incubation period—The time between exposure to disease and the onset of the disease

Infectious agents—Organisms that cause infection

Intercostal space—The space between ribs

IO—Intraosseous

IP—Intraperitoneal

IV—Intravenous

Jaundice—A condition in which the waste product bilirubin builds up in the body and causes the yellowing of mucus membranes within the body

Jugular vein—A vein that returns blood from the head and neck to the heart

Keel—Bony ridge on the sternum of birds where the flight muscles attach

Keratin—A tough, waterproof protein that makes up scales, beaks, and claws of animals

Keratitis—Inflammation of the cornea of the eye

kg, mg, g or gm—kilogram, milligram, gram

kl, ml, l—kiloliter, milliliter, liter

kPa—Kilopascal

Laryngoscope—An instrument that aids in the insertion of an endotracheal tube

Lateral—Located away from the center of the body

Leukopenia—A condition that causes a below-average number of white blood cells

Lichenification—Thickening or hardening of the skin

Lipids—Various substances, such as fats, that are soluble in nonpolar organic solvents and insoluble in water

Lymph nodes—Small masses of tissue within the lymphatic system that contain white blood cells and filter bacteria and foreign particles from the lymphatic system

Malignant—Tendency of a condition to become progressively worse

Mandible—The bone of the lower jaw

MAP—Mean arterial pressure

Masticate—To chew or crush

Mastitis—Inflammation of the mammary glands

Maxilla—The bone of the upper jaw

Medial—Toward the midline of the body

Monogastric—Having a simple, single-chambered stomach

Necrosis—The death and breakdown of cells

Neuropathy—Abnormal function of the nerves

Neuter—Sterilization of a male animal

Nocturnal—Of or relating to the night time

NPO—Nothing by mouth

O.D.—Right eye

OFD—Object film distance

Oliguria—The excretion of less urine than normal

Omnivore—Animal that eats both meat and plants

Opioid—Drug that has effects similar to opium

Orchiectomy—Surgical removal of a male animal's testes

O.S.—Left eye

O.U.—Both eyes

Oviposition—The act of laying eggs

Palpation—To examine with the hands or fingers

Pancreatitis—Inflammation of the pancreas

Parturition—The act of giving birth

PCV—Pack cell volume

Peritonitis—Inflammation of the lining of the abdomen

Pica—A condition that causes the chronic eating of items that are not normally eaten

Plaque—A buildup on the teeth

Platelets—Cellular components of the blood that help clots to form

PO—Per os, by mouth

Polyuria—Excessive urination

Posterior—Located behind or toward the rear

PRN—As needed

Proximal—Located or situated toward the body

Pruritus—Itching

psi—Pounds per square inch

Pyometra—Disease of the uterus characterized by the accumulation of pus.

q.d.—Once a day

q.i.d.—Four times a day (every six hours)

Radiograph—An X-ray

RBC—Red blood cell

Red blood cell (RBC)—A blood cell that contains hemoglobin and is responsible for the transport of oxygen and carbon dioxide

Regurgitation—The act of expelling food from the esophagus

Ruminant—An herbivore that has a complex, four-chambered stomach, such as cattle, goats, and sheep

Sarcoptic mange—Skin disease caused by the bite of a parasitic mite that causes extreme itching and hair loss

SC or SQ—Subcutaneous

Sepsis—The presence of toxins in the blood or other tissues

s.i.d.—Once a day

SID—Source image distance

Skin cytology—Examination of a skin scraping or material from swabbing the skin

Spay—Sterilization of a female animal

Spirochete—A long, slender bacteria that assumes a spiral shape

Squamate—Scaly-bodied reptile

Supraventricular tachycardia—A condition that causes the heart to beat very rapidly because of signals coming from the atria or near the junction of the atria with the ventricles

Syncope—Temporary loss of consciousness

Thrombocytopenia—A lower than normal number of platelets in the blood

t.i.d.—Three times a day (every 8 hours)

Titer—A measurement of the amount of antibodies in the blood

U/A—Urinalysis

Urticaria—The development of hives

Uveitis—Inflammation of the uvea or middle, vascular portion of the eye

Vasculitis—Inflammation of blood vessels

Ventral—Located toward the belly or floor

Vertebrate—Animal with a vertebral column (or spine)

Whelping—The act of giving birth in dogs

White blood cell (WBC)—Blood cell lacking hemoglobin that helps protect the body from infection

Recommended Resources

Veterinary technicians and other professionals in veterinary medicine should be aware of the important professional organizations related to their field. The resources listed in this appendix can be accessed to gain current information about the field of veterinary medicine and can be contacted about any professional questions or concerns.

The following list contains only a fraction of the resources available to veterinary technicians. If you need further information from a source that is not included in this list, visit the American Veterinary Medical Association's Web site for a more comprehensive list of resources.

A

Academy of Internal Medicine for Veterinary Technicians
P.O. Box 75221
Seattle, Washington 98175-0221
Web site: www.aimvt.com

Academy of Veterinary Behavior Technicians
Web site: www.avbt.net

Academy of Veterinary Dental Technicians
Web site: www.avdt.us

Academy of Veterinary Emergency and Critical Care Technicians
Web site: www.avecct.org

Academy of Veterinary Surgical Technicians
Web site: www.avst-vts.org

Academy of Veterinary Technician Anesthetists
Web site: www.avta-vts.org

Academy of Veterinary Technicians in Clinical Practice
Web site: www.avtcp.org

Academy of Veterinary Zoological Medicine
Web site: www.avzmt.org

American Association of Equine Veterinary Technicians and Assistants
Web site: www.aaevt.org

American Association for Laboratory Animal Science
9190 Crestwyn Hills Drive
Memphis, Tennessee 38125-8538
Phone: 901-754-8620
Fax: 901-753-0046
Web site: www.aalas.org

American Association of Veterinary Medical Colleges
1101 Vermont Avenue, NW
Suite 301
Washington, D.C. 20005
Phone: 202-371-9195
Fax: 202-842-0773
Web site: www.aavmc.org

American College of Veterinary Anesthesiologists
P.O. Box 1100
Middleburg, Virginia 20118
Web site: www.acva.org

American College of Veterinary Preventative Medicine
2150 Fairview Circle
Garden Ridge, Texas 78266
Phone: 210-382-5400
Web site: www.acvpm.org

American College of Veterinary Surgeons
19785 Crystal Rock Drive
Suite 305
Germantown, Maryland 20874
Phone: 301-916-0200
           877-217-2287 (toll-free)
Fax: 301-916-2287
Web site: www.acvs.org

American Dairy Science Association
2441 Village Green Place
Champaign, Illinois 6182
Phone: 217-356-5146
Fax: 217-398-4119
Web site: www.adsa.org

American Humane Association
63 Inverness Drive E
Englewood, Colorado 80112
Phone: 303-792-9900
           800-227-4645 (toll-free)
Fax: 303-792-5333
Web site: www.americanhumane.org

American Kennel Club
8051 Arco Corporate Drive
Suite 100
Raleigh, North Carolina 27617
Phone: 919-233-9767
Web site: www.akc.org

American Society for the Prevention of Cruelty to Animals
424 East 92nd Street
New York, New York 10128
Phone: 212-876-7700
Web site: www.aspca.org

American Veterinary Medical Association
1931 N. Meacham Road
Suite 100
Schaumburg, Illinois 60173
Phone: 800-248-2862 (toll-free)
Fax: 847-925-1329
Web site: www.avma.org

Animal Agriculture Alliance
P.O. Box 9522
Arlington, Virginia 22209
Phone: 703-562-5160
Web site: www.animalagalliance.org

Animal Behavior Society
Indiana University
402 N. Park Avenue
Bloomington, Indiana 47408
Phone: 812-856-5541
Fax: 812-856-5542
Web site: http://animalbehaviorsociety.org

Animal Welfare Institute
900 Pennsylvania Avenue, SE
Washington, D.C. 20003
Phone: 202-337-2332
Web site: www.awionline.org

Association for Women Veterinarians Foundation
2525 McGaw Avenue
Irvine, California 92614
Phone: 949-660-2412
Web site: www.womenveterinarians.org

Association of Zoos and Aquariums
8403 Colesville Road
Suite 710
Silver Spring, Maryland 20910
Phone: 301-562-0777
Fax: 301-562-0888
Web site: www.aza.org

C

Center for Veterinary Medicine
7519 Standish Place
HFV-12
Rockville, Maryland 20855
Phone: 240-276-9300
Web site: www.fda.gov/AnimalVeterinary/

Christian Veterinary Mission
19303 Fremont Avenue N
Seattle, Washington 98133
Phone: 206-546-7569
Fax: 206-546-7458
Web site: www.cvmusa.org

Conservation Breeding Specialist Group
12101 Johnny Cake Ridge Road
Apple Valley, Minnesota 55124
Phone: 952-997-9800
Fax: 952-997-9803
Web site: www.cbsg.org/cbsg

D

Delta Society
875 124th Avenue
Suite 101
Bellevue, Washington 98005
Web site: www.deltasociety.org

E

Entomological Society of America
10001 Derekwood Lane
Suite 100
Lanham, Maryland 20706
Phone: 301-731-4535
Fax: 301-731-4538
Web site: www.entsoc.org

F

Foundation for Biomedical Research
818 Connecticut Avenue, NW
Suite 900
Washington, D.C. 20006
Phone: 202-457-0654
Fax: 202-457-0659
Web site: www.fbresearch.org

G

Guide Dog Foundation for the Blind, Inc.
371 East Jericho Turnpike
Smithtown, New York 11787
Phone: 800-548-4337 (toll-free)
Web site: www.guidedog.org

H

Health and Science Communications Association
39 Wedgewood Drive
Suite A
Jewett City, Connecticut 06351
Phone: 860-376-5915
Web site: www.hesca.org

I

International Veterinary Academy of Pain Management
618 Church Street
Suite 220
Nashville, Tennessee 37219
Phone: 615-301-3040
Fax: 615-254-7047
Web site: www.ivapm.org

L

Lesbian and Gay Veterinary Medical Association
584 Castro Street
Suite 492
San Francisco, California 94114
Fax: 503-213-8749
Web site: www.lgvma.org

M

Morris Animal Foundation
10200 East Girard Avenue
Suite B430
Denver, Colorado 80231
Phone: 303-790-2345
             800-243-2345 (toll-free)
Fax: 303-790-4066
Web site: www.morrisanimalfoundation.org

N

National Animal Interest Alliance
P.O. Box 66579
Portland, Oregon 97290
Phone: 503-761-1139
Web site: www.naiaonline.org

National Association of Animal Breeders
P.O. Box 1033
Columbia, Missouri 65205
Phone: 573-445-4406
Fax: 573-446-2279
Web site: www.naab-css.org

National Association of Veterinary Technicians in America (NAVTA)
1666 K Street, NW
Suite 260
Washington, D.C. 20006
Phone: 703-40-8737
Fax: 202-49-8560
Web site: www.navta.net

National Farmers Union
20 F Street, NW
Suite 300
Washington, D.C. 20001
Phone: 202-554-1600
Web site: www.nfu.org

O

Orthopedic Foundation for Animals
2300 East Nifong Boulevard
Columbia, Missouri 65201
Phone: 573-442-0418
Fax: 573-875-5073
Web site: www.offa.org

P

Pet Industry Joint Advisory Council
1140 19th Street, NW
Suite 300
Washington, D.C. 20036
Phone: 202-452-1525
               800-553-7387 (toll-free)
Fax: 202-452-1516
Web site: www.pijac.org

S

Society for Marine Mammalogy
41 Green Acres Road
Hartford, Maine 04220
Phone: 207-597-2333
Web site: www.marinemammalscience.org

Society for Tropical Veterinary Medicine
Oklahoma State University
250 McElroy Hall
Stillwater, Oklahoma 74078
Phone: 405-744-6726
Web site: www.soctropvetmed.org

T

Tuscon Herpetological Society
P.O. Box 709
Tucson, Arizona 85702
Web site: http://cfa.arizona.edu

U

United States Animal Health Association
P.O. Box 8805
St. Joseph, Missouri 64508
Phone: 816-671-1144
Fax: 816-671-1201
Web site: www.usaha.org

V

Veterinary Cancer Society
P.O. Box 1763
Spring Valley, California 91979
Phone: 619-741-2210
Fax: 619-741-1117
Web site: www.vetcancersociety.org

Veterinary Information Network
777 W. Covell Boulevard
Davis, California 95616
Phone: 530-756-4881
               800-700-4636 (toll-free)
Fax: 530-756-6035
Web site: www.vin.com

W

World Aquaculture Society
Louisiana State University
143 J. M. Parker Coliseum
Baton Rouge, Louisiana 70803
Phone: 225-578-3137
Fax: 225-578-3493
Web site: www.was.org

SPECIAL ADVERTISING SECTION

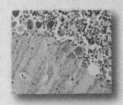
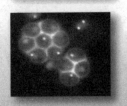
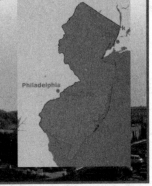
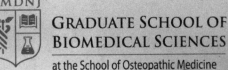

Learn from a National Leader in
Population Health

Jefferson School of Population Health

- **Master of Public Health (MPH); CEPH accredited**

- **PhD in Population Health Sciences**

Online programs

- **Master of Science in Health Policy (MS-HP)**

- **Master of Science in Healthcare Quality and Safety (MS-HQS)**

- **Master of Science in Chronic Care Management (MS-CCM)**

- **Certificates in Public Health, Health Policy, Healthcare Quality and Safety, Chronic Care Management**

Population health – putting health and health care together

215-503-0174

www.jefferson.edu/population_health/ads.cfm

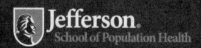

Jefferson.
School of Population Health

THOMAS JEFFERSON UNIVERSITY

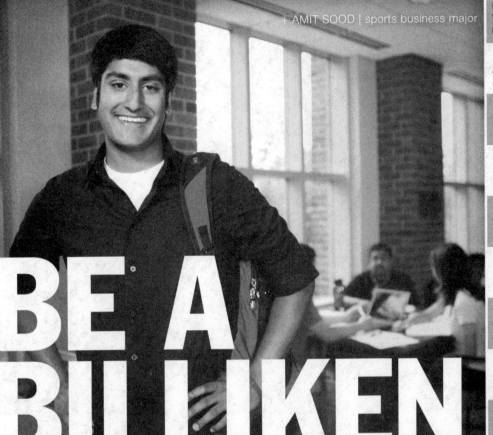

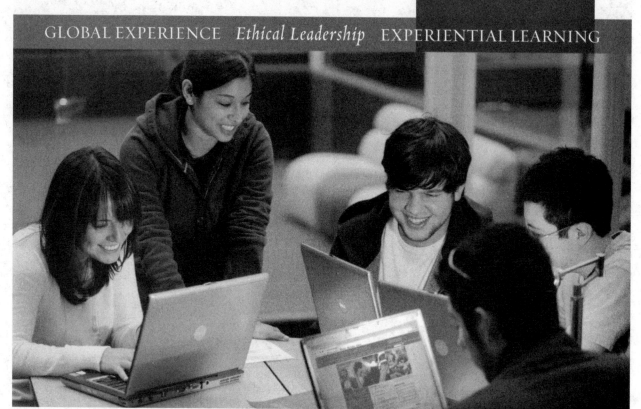

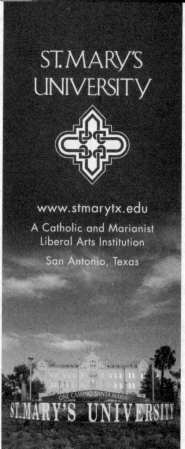

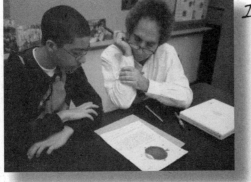
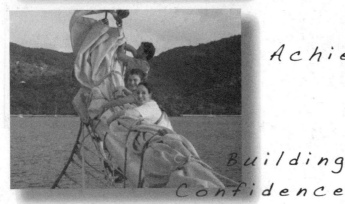
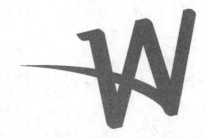